Sociology of Health in a Dalit Community

Sociology of Health in a Dalit Community:

Axes of Exclusion of Hadis

By

K. M. Ziyauddin

Cambridge Scholars Publishing

Sociology of Health in a Dalit Community: Axes of Exclusion of Hadis

By K. M. Ziyauddin

This book first published 2024

Cambridge Scholars Publishing

Lady Stephenson Library, Newcastle upon Tyne, NE6 2PA, UK

British Library Cataloguing in Publication Data
A catalogue record for this book is available from the British Library

ISBN (10): 1-4438-4003-3
ISBN (13): 978-1-4438-4003-3

For

Abbu and Ammi

And all my field respondents including Gandhi Hadi

CONTENTS

ACKNOWLEDGEMENTS

The author would like to thank Sanghmitra S. Acharya for her help and encouragement while writing this book. The dissertation's constraints were overcome thanks to my insightful and impromptu conversations with her. It is a wonderful occasion to thank her for her steady, affectionate, and academic encouragement throughout the last two decades. The author's dedication to helping underrepresented groups grew more robust as a result of this period. Sincere thanks are also due to Ghanshyam Shah, who provided invaluable assistance before and after the dissertation's submission at JNU's Centre for Social Medicine and Community Health in New Delhi.

Maintaining the dual identities of a social anthropologist and a public health professional while working in the field was challenging. All of this, however, was simplified by the centre's welcoming atmosphere. While at the Centre of Social Medicine and Community Health at Jawaharlal Nehru University, Rama V. Baru was an invaluable source of encouragement and insight. The notion of a public health viewpoint and health care services was formed through open and close communication with all the instructors at the centre and school. It is also important to highlight the helpfulness of the centre's library employees. Tulsi Patel, Anand Kumar, Abhijit Dasgupta, Mohammad Talib, Abdul Matin, Arvinder Ansari, Mohammad Akram, and many more have tremendously influenced me during my education and continue to do so now.

My education at Jamia Millia Islamia, Jawaharlal Nehru University, and the Delhi School of Economics at the University of Delhi gave me the tools to approach my research with sensitivity and dedication. Frequently communicating with many of my professors and friends across all three institutions inspired the current volume. I am profoundly grateful to each of them and to the librarians at all three institutions.

The study on Hadis was one of the most challenging projects I've ever worked on (Navin and Matthew are very knowledgeable in my subject). For my dissertation, though, I doubled down on investigating this same social class. The training I obtained under Tulsi Patel, my leader and true mentor at the Delhi School of Economics, University of Delhi, completely reshaped the fieldwork and method of my study. This university shaped my worldview into that of a social anthropologist and compelled me to undertake extensive fieldwork. I owe her an outstanding debt of gratitude for the research potential she sparked in me, and I could ask for nothing more than to have her constant mentoring from beginning to end in all of my research and education. I'd also like to extend my gratitude to everyone who assisted me in any way during my fieldwork, including V. K. Singh (IAS), Dr Mandal, Rajesh, Aijaz, Gandhi, Mantu, Santu, Dilip, and all the responders to Hadi Cooli, who is still a wonderful guy to this day. Because the doctorate thesis explores disease and health among Dalits from a fresh and different angle, I am pleased to publish the M.Phil. dissertation in book form. The Hadi caste in India is the subject of this first-ever academic investigation.

I want to thank the Foundation for Social Care, which generously supported my M.Phil. programme through a merit-based scholarship.

Many others, including Rajan, Shashi, Mathew, Navin, Vinod, Uddhab, Farooque, Moin, Shattarupa, Santhosh, Retheesh, Smita, and Anil, to name a few, and Aboobakar Siddique, IAS, and Gulam Samdani, SDO, deserve credit for helping me get the resources and access I needed to do my fieldwork. Many of my colleagues at Urdu University and the University of Hyderabad's Institute for the Study of Social Exclusion and Inclusive Policy provided invaluable insight and advice. The list continues with names like Kancha Ilaiah, Abdul Matin, Farida Siddiqui, Afroz Alam, Shahid, Nageshwara, Abdul Thaha, Salma Farooqui, Salil Kader, Anil, Ashwani, H. Y. Siddiqui, E. Kasi, G. Nagaraju, Saheed, and Shahid Raza. Without meeting with some old friends and acquaintances from Delhi, my time in Hyderabad would have been much lonelier. Friends like Jamaluddin Khan, Firoze Alam, Qaiser, Athar, Imtiyaz, Kashif, Obaid, and notably Fahatullah Beig are solely responsible for instilling in me the curiosity and enthusiasm for novel ideas, cuisine, history, and culture that allowed me to establish myself in Hyderabad securely. Deccan's fundamentally multiethnic civilisation gives a challenge to the field of research and happiness to the people; therefore, its residents' sense of calm and serenity shouldn't come as much of a surprise. I'd also like to express my appreciation to everyone on my CSSEIP team who has assisted me in any way.

The CSSEIP and Central Library librarians' collaboration was invaluable in this research. Special thanks to respected teacher and outstanding scholar Prof. Syed Ainul Hasan, Vice Chancellor of Maulana Azad National Urdu University, for providing us with the academic leadership we desperately needed. Lastly, I'd like to thank my DSW colleagues, Syed Aleem Ashraf Jaisi, Sami Siddiqui, Ismath, Jameel, and Jarrar, for helping me maintain my academic enthusiasm despite our hectic schedules throughout COVID-19. My wife, Hena Kauser, back home in Hyderabad, deserves my most incredible gratitude for her unending support of this research and all my other academic endeavours. She relieves the burden of time's relentless demands. She's been a tremendous assistance to me while I've penned this massive work, mainly since completing her PhD thesis taught her the value of patience. Having my kids Adifaah Ziya (Falak) and Khwaja Aaraf around with their bright, eye-catching antics energised me during long studying periods at home during the pandemic. The siblings in my house—Tabrez, Naghma, Afroz, Afsar, and Bushra—are always interested in what I'm up to and want to see my latest creations. I hope people find some pleasure in this publication. They (my uncle Khwaja Ekram at JNU and the rest of my family) have earned this moment of celebration, and I am grateful to be able to enjoy it with them.

I appreciate Elisabeth's careful editing, the hard work of the entire CSP team, especially Amanda Miller and Rebecca, and the fruitful discussions we had on the content and language. For their early help with some light editing of the book, I also have to thank Subrata and Mudassir Nazr.

I am grateful to my parents and my sweetest Daadi Amma (who passed during COVID-19), who was there for me through thick and thin till she passed away. My gratitude will never be enough, but I hope they will always consider me unique. Dadi Amma, wherever she may be, would be pleased to hear that this book is finally being published.

2024
K. M. ZIYAUDDIN

FOREWORD

This book is a pioneering work exploring the issues of health concern of the *Hadis* and *Bauris* – two communities that have been traditionally engaged in the cleaning occupation. The book delves into the health problems that have plagued certain Dalit communities in India for years. While there is vast literature existing on workers in construction, garment, and even hazardous industries, very little is evident for the workers who ransom their lives and health, for sure, to provide cleanliness to the living spaces of people who label them as unclean and often 'polluted'. A sincere endeavour to trace the social history of these communities and connect it with the current public health system is visible through the work in different chapters. The book has very neatly established the relationship between caste-based occupations led exclusion of this group of people (*Hadis* and *Bauri*), and the consequent denial of opportunities which have led to their poor education, skill, and economic potential. The social, cultural, political, and economic exclusion of these people exists in many forms and nature. The book captures these through experiential evidence and reflects on the inequalities which have existed historically on varied axes of social, economic, political, and cultural indicators.

This book is a timely contribution to the research on caste and occupation inter-linkages. It is also well-timed to commemorate the 125th birth anniversary of Dr BR Ambedkar, whose untiring efforts have ensured some affirmative action for the underprivileged people through constitutional safeguards in inclusive development processes. At present, when a lot of emphases are being given on cleanliness and sanitation, almost in the mission mode, the present book is a strong comment on the status of those who ensure the provisioning of clean and sanitised surroundings. A socially conscious readership will welcome this book, for it triggers the minds of all those who are concerned with social equality, the environment, and the upkeep of constitutional safeguards.

January 2024

(Sanghmitra S Acharya)
Professor, Centre of Social Medicine and Community Health
School of Social Sciences, Jawaharlal Nehru University, New Delhi
Former Director, Indian Institute of Dalit Studies, New Delhi

PREFACE

This book elaborates on aspects of the health situation of certain Dalit communities (in India) who have suffered and have been suffering for generations. The case is given for the Hadi caste with a focus on Bauris as a brief point of reference. The book is primarily based on the fieldwork conducted as a part of my M. Phil programme at the Centre of Social Medicine and Community Health at Jawaharlal Nehru University, New Delhi. The newest data has been systematically integrated into the present book, collected during the field visits conducted over the past few years.

Where necessary, the experience of the researcher in the field is added to elaborate on the Bauris and their life at the margin. The chapters not only describe the health conditions in detail but also how a myriad of experiences shapes the community as a caste group and as "untouchables". The state of Jharkhand has been home to the Bauri caste as one of the largest Dalit communities, and they comprise a small chunk of the population among the other Scheduled Caste groups there. Occupation, customs, rituals, social interaction, and many more aspects have been covered in the book to enhance the generalisable capability of the present work.

The book also looks into the health of the studied population as seen from a public health perspective. The traditional occupation of the *Hadis* helps us to build an understanding of the accessibility and availability of health services in India. The experiences of illness do not describe the reality; rather, a long-term negative impact occurs due to community experiences at health care centres and hospitals. The elaboration on these Dalit castes reflects the historically committed mistake within the larger spectrum of the Hindu caste society in India. The socio-religious sanctity of the unequal and discriminatory social arrangement for different occupations changed the course of Indian social life. How occupation and caste can become the only identities of a social group, which in turn leads to several consequences affecting the basic fundamental rights of the deprived populations, is also discussed here in this book.

It is important to examine caste and occupation-based exclusion, but the systemic and constitutive exclusion carried for years requires serious examination in itself. This is experienced on social, cultural, political and economic fronts because exclusion exists in complex forms and is multi-dimensional. Interestingly, the book attempts to analyse also the problem of being a field researcher and provides an account of researchers' experiences in this particular domain. This will help all research bases and initiatives focusing on caste and occupation as variables.

The multidisciplinary nature of the book will be helpful for students and researchers of sociology, anthropology, public health, historical and political studies, demography, social work, and gender studies, social exclusion in particular and humanities in general.

K.M. ZIYAUDDIN
Hyderabad, India

CHAPTER ONE

SOCIOLOGY OF HEALTH AND SOCIAL EXCLUSION

1. Background

The heterogeneity of Indian society and the Indian state remains a silent reality of contemporary society. Nevertheless, this cannot be accepted as recognition of the state's achievement; instead, the masked brutalities of lost and damaged lives are the crude reality of excluded groups in India and demand a scientific inquiry to understand the problem. The majority of sufferers belong to the Scheduled Castes, referred to as Dalits in the present writings. The state has grossly maltreated these people in critical health, nutrition, public safety, assurance of employment, and education.

This gross negligence appears as a point of social exclusion. The most discussed concern about the caste system remains its influence in every sphere of life, health, education, employment. Dalits have been seriously affected in terms of health and quality of life. The experience of untouchability did not vanish from the Dalits' social context and still appears in debates on the sociology of health. The larger picture in this book is to understand the sociological dimensions of Dalits' health and approach the field from public health questions.

Another point of social exclusion is seen in census enumerations. Even the Census of India enumerated and classified only the untouchable caste of the Hindu religion and not of the other religions practised in India such as Sikhism, Christianity, and Buddhism. In particular, untouchable castes that converted to Christianity or Sikhism, and even in limited context amongst Indian Muslims, continued to be untouchable despite their change in religion.

Without any inhibitions, studies proved (such as Shah et al., 2002) that caste oppression, particularly in rural areas, remains acute; also, infringements of caste rules on moral and sexual conduct have been known to lead to the death of those who dare to transgress and break these rules. The unwritten rule of touchability is still the standard norm experienced in the lives of both rural and urban Dalits. Despite promises made by ruling parties, abuse of women continues virtually unchecked. It is a severe problem for Dalit women in India.

The debate on Dalits' health and especially of those engaged in "unclean" or "polluted" occupations emerges when factoring in the context of other aspects of their life and examining caste-based social surroundings they live in.

The concepts of equal and free education, food and shelter, and health facilities have been repeatedly designed in every five-year plan since independence. According to the 1991 census of India, however, this appears to remain a distant dream for the 138 million people belonging to Scheduled Castes (SCs) that constitute 16.48 per cent of the country's total population (Shah 2001) continues further. Thus, it becomes vital to understand their socio-economic conditions, regional distribution, perception of health and access to various resources, including health care. In this regard, a very distinct observation is that most of the menial and low-ranking jobs are either reserved for or occupied by Dalits, i.e. very few occupy high-ranking jobs profile. More often than not, the shares of the reserved posts are not fulfilled in various state departments and institutions. Why is it that advertisements are constantly put out for low-ranking jobs? The reason varies from "non-availability" of a suitable candidate or popularly known as "Not Found Suitable (NFS)" to actual lower levels of education and general awareness that restricts the *Dalits* from availing the opportunities.

Persistent negligence has affected the health status of Dalits in India. The present book is neither about the history of Dalits nor about the exploitation and discrimination do they face. Already there are a few facts and realities of Indian society. Before we discuss the basic concept of Dalits' health status, it will be necessary to briefly trace the history of the caste system in India and its different faces since its inception. Without examining the caste system as unique to the Hindu social system, it may be difficult to understand the various factors related to the life under Hindu social structure. The "one-man theory" based on Shastras has not served to launch a dialogue and conversation among Indian social scientists; however, a few western scholars, probably not much disposed of/inclined to hero-worship, have tried to provide a scientific explanation. The "nuclei around which have "formed" the various castes in India are (1) Occupation; (2) Survival of tribal organisations, (3) the rise of new belief, (4) cross-breeding and (5) migration" (WSBRA 1979).

In Indian society, socio-community and spiritual and traditional occupations override all class factors. In contrast, in western countries, the significant factors that determine the different strata of the society, viz. wealth, education and vocation, are fluid and Catholic (general or universal) and tend to modify the rigidity of birth and hereditary position.

Understanding the sociology of health in a Dalit community is important while examining the interactions with doctors, health professionals, and patients at present. It was a different context when sociology of health emerged in the 1950s as a specialised area of sociology. However, the continued increase in the narrative in illness and health has made this area of research much more serious and significant. The exclusion of a Dalit community is reflected when one deals with power issues between doctors and patients, between health and the state (Nagla, 2014). The discussions on the questions to access and utilisation of health care and the kind of discriminatory experiences of Dalits bring the sociological importance on health and health care. Several studies have brought the core value of the discipline in contrast to purely non-sociological studies. We have a few references to benefit from the ethnographic details on fever in Kerala (George, 2014), Prasad's (2014) study on Malaria, among other studies.

1.1 Class and Class Inequality

Social inequality is a universal phenomenon. It either exists in the form of a hierarchy of groups or individuals, or it may exist without the creation of a hierarchy. In the former case, it is called social hierarchy, while in the latter case, it is known as social differentiation. On the other hand, if social inequality manifests itself in the form of a hierarchy involving a ranking of groups, then it is known as social stratification. Thus, social stratification is a particular case of social inequality. The different forms of social inequality generate tensions and create conflict in the basic fabric of any society. However, the existence of class in society helps to function into the evolving mechanisms, and they decrease the rigidity of caste hierarchy based on birth and occupation.

Further, Gupta (1991) adds that "class is a system of stratification that is economic in character". His commentary on the caste system with its myriad forms of superordination and subordination, its many customs and taboos, perhaps most responsible for conferring on India. But this is not all. India is also economically stratified.

In the context of class formation, Karl Marx talks about the different stages in the history of society. Marx views class as a group whose members share the same relationship to the forces of production. He argues that in every society, there are two groups: the "haves" and the "have nots". In his important book, Benedix and Lipset (1996) state that, "a social class in Marx's terms is an aggregate of persons who perform the same function in the organisation of production". Like Marx, Weber also sees class in economic terms. He argues that classes develop in market economies in which individuals compete for personal gain and benefits. He defines it as a "group of individuals who share a similar position in the market economy and by that fact receives economic rewards". Thus, in Weber's terminology, a person's class situation is his "market situation". Hence, those who share a similar class situation also share similar life chances.

Now, if we look at the post-independence era in India, planned development has been an important model for the benefit of all classes but has only benefited certain classes, leaving aside the groups of deprived and weaker castes. The "trickle-down" theory was adopted by the Indian government to provide opportunities across caste and class, but at the grassroots level, it seems to have failed. In fact, the "trickle-down" process has narrowed connotation for a similar reason. It means that as a result of macro processes, such as economic growth, certain benefits may accrue to the downtrodden, who may be a little better off than before. But it may not reduce the differences between those who possess the power of social, economic, and political influence and others who don't deserve these. The trickle-down theory "does not suggest empowerment and achievement of equity" (Nadkarni 1997). But the process created a huge gap between the classes and castes.

Beteille (1977) provides a new paradigm to understand the historical distinction of inequality, "neutral inequalities" among men and inequalities among "their conditions of existence". Now the discussion will move on to examine the interdependent variables such as caste.

1.2 Genesis of the Caste System in India

The Indian concept of caste is different from those of other countries where it exists. The complexities surrounding the concept of caste and its origin are not new to us. Most of the theories which explain its origin have not been able to prove and satisfy the emerging queries because each theory has its causal explanation. There are few approaches to understanding the origin of caste in India.

One of the most common words for the genus in most Indian languages, "*Jati*," is derived from an Indo-European verbal root meaning "genesis," "origin," or "birth". It is applied to any species of living things, including gods and humans. Among humans, *Jati* can designate a distinct sex, a race, a caste or a tribe; a family, a lineage, or a clan; an ethnic group, a regional population, the followers of an occupation or a religion, or a nation (Encyclopaedia of Britannica 1969).

The fate of the history of caste and *Jati* is manifested in the Vedic Age (1750-500 BE) and can be traced throughout history. Gupta (2000) argued that in "realities there are thousands of *Jati*s that caste injunctions on marriage, occupation and social relations are conducted". It is essential to understand the genesis of caste in the Varna system in India. *Varnas* is the dominant theoretical explanation (Gupta 1991). *Brahmins, Kshatriyas, Vaishyas,* and *Shudras* (Jhunjhunwala 1999), were all created by *Varna* from the *Lord Brahma's* mouth, arm, thigh, and soul, respectively. Each group consists of different castes, and they are restricted in terms of food, marriage, rituals, and festivals.

The four-fold division of the caste system has resulted in sharp distinction, and thus it is a strong expression of social stratification. Marriott (1973) "sketches the idea regarding caste and its functions through the ethnographic approach".

1.3 The Question of Caste and Class

The uniqueness of Indian society lies in the caste system, which has managed to maintain the hierarchical system very smoothly, but this fact is the crudest form of social exclusion. For quite a long time, it has been argued that this is the best functioning of social activities. Caste provides a critical paradigm to locate an individual and a group's social, political, economic, and religious life. The attempt in this volume is not to portray caste as the most functional system instead to critically question and understand the entire discourse that has perpetuated the caste system even today. Undoubtedly, the changing global economy has made the process of change faster and created a new consumer class, where the uniqueness of caste is being diluted into class. As an institution of considerable internal complexity, caste has been oversimplified by those seeking an ideal rigid hierarchical social stratification based on extremely closed criteria based on an individual's birth in a family. Consequently, we see that the complexities of the caste system have remained troublesome to the entire Dalit population and other marginalised groups.

According to Andre Beteille (1997), "Caste is a small and named group of persons characterised by endogamy, hereditary membership, and a specific lifestyle that sometimes includes the pursuit by the tradition of a particular occupation and is usually associated with a more or less distinct ritual status in a hierarchical system, based on the concept of purity and pollution,"

Caste structure has its distinct features compared with other forms of social structure. Ghurye (1969) has divided these features into six categories—choice of occupation is not an option for an individual or family belonging to the Dalit caste. The basis of the conceptualisation of any particular occupation has been pollution and, in consequence, how pollution is linked to certain caste groups. Beteille (1997) cited, from *Homo Hierarchicus: the Caste System and Its Implications* (Louis Dumont, 1980), that "the principle of purity provides the key to the understanding of evaluation and hierarchy in Indian society. Objects, beings, events, places, conditions, individuals and groups are all invested with varying degrees of purity-impurity and are arranged in hierarchical orders". This illustrates the status of groups fallen into the polluted category due to hereditary occupational associations such as manual scavenging.

The *Varna* System provides the system of values; the *Jati* is the functional organisation and practice. *Jati*s may seek promotion within the caste hierarchy by adopting the practices of the higher *Varna*, which can result in promotion within their *Varna* but not between *Varna*, a process known as Sanskritization. In a nutshell, "Sanskritization" is "the process of adopting the practises, rituals, food habits, and dress styles of the Sanskrits or upper castes." The term was coined to describe the changes occurring in a village among the Coorgs in Mysore.

Since independence in 1947, India has attempted to break down caste divisions, though, in practice, caste retains a vital role in a social structure. Some sociologists have attempted, amid controversy, to extend the term beyond Indian society and apply it (not only) to the analysis of the South African system of Apartheid, but even to the system of the United States during the twentieth century. The period after the assassination of King Martin Luther witnessed a phase of the civil rights movement taking an aggressive phase in America. Andrews (1997), in his study on the impact of social movements on the political processes, does identify the underlying reasons that gave support base to the civil rights movement in America. Some of the legislations of the American government paved the path of the civil rights movement and their demands. From 1954 to 1968, American society gave rise to the demands of civil rights within society, and it was also directly linked to the U.S. Supreme Court's decision on Brown vs Board of Education, culminating after the assassination of King Luther. The same period also had barriers towards blacks from realising first-class citizenship in America. In most studies, it was deliberated how the civil rights movement made (Luders, 2010) its presence, showed the effectiveness and tried to measure the presence of racial groups in the neighbourhood. However, it did not understand why people were racially segregated USA. However, the recent efforts as a new approach "based on growth mixture models can be used to identify patterns of racial change that distinguish between durable integration and gradual racial succession. The detailed writings of Michael and Warkentein (2016) on 'The Fragmented Evolution of Racial Integration since the Civil Rights Movement' talk about the mixture models, a helpful approach to identify the various patterns of racial change. One does find the typical trace of neighbourhood racial change found among several groups, namely blacks, whites, Latinos, and Asians, from 1970 to 2010. This pattern is seen in the New York, Los Angeles, Chicago, and Houston Metropolitan areas showing nominally integrated neighbourhoods that have experienced a gradual succession. The effort in this section is to precisely refer to the changes that took after the civil rights movement in America, which has also given some direction to future studies on Dalits in India.

However, in India, the birth-based ascribed status of all those in Hindu religions has a strong impact that governs the everyday life of each individual on the line of caste principles, which was regressive. It was used to exploit already deprived classes in a very systematic way, in all aspects: socially, economically, and politically and had no other avenues that could help the lower castes to escape from their traditional identity throughout Indian history.

2. Dalits, their Evolution and Background

The oppression and exploitation of Dalits as untouchables has been a phenomenal practice, dating almost three thousand years. They are the people who have to do menial and degrading jobs. They are segregated in all spheres of social life: places of worship, education, housing, land ownership, use of common wells, roads, public transport, and accessibility of health services. All this suggests that it is imperative to measure the socio-economic factors which have forced Dalits to stay in a condition of exploitation.

The question of the Dalit caste is susceptible and carries much debate in itself. Why are Dalits “Dalit”? Who are the people being deprived of social status in terms of having a high ranking in the social order? The pertinent question raised by Webster (1994) about the ancestors of today’s Dalits; how and why did they become untouchables in the particular religious framework are significant. It is also essential to understand how academia understands the ruptured social fabric based on caste hierarchy. There are occasions to put the question of Dalit identity at the forefront of the mainstream debate among scholars is utilised.

Dalits are defined as “downtrodden, deprived and exploited”. They are discriminated against socially, economically, and politically. The most frustrating obstacles in their life are the concepts of “purity” and “pollution”. They symbolise “pollution” and thus “untouchability”. Theological explanations generally do not provide or accommodate any space to scientificity because theology believes that one must surrender before the unseen fact. At the same time, science needs logical explanations and applicability in contemporary periods or societies on vivid and different grounds (Massey 1997).

According to the code of Manusmirti (1500 BC), the untouchables were not supposed to own property. Manu states that concerning the Shudra or servant castes, he should not amass wealth even if he has the ability for a servant who has amassed some wealth to annoy the priests. The social, political, and economic discrimination based on religious sanction was glorified and explained through the theory of divinity and Karma. The origin of the caste system is in the *Varnasram* Dharma, the division of society into four *Varna*s (four castes), viz. Brahmin, Kshatriya, Vaishya, and Shudra. It is believed that for the world’s prosperity, the Creator created four *Varna*s from different parts of the body. He created Brahmins with Gayatri (metre-Vedic meter refers to the poetic meter used in the Vedic literature), the Kshatriyas with trishubh (tripudium), the Vaishyas with Jagati, and the Shudras without any metre (The Bhopal Document 2002).

The first three *Varna*s are twice-born (dwiji). The first birth is from the mother and the second from the investiture with the sacred thread. In the second birth, Savitri is the mother, and the teacher is the father because he gives instructions in the *Vedas*. Therefore, the first three *Varna*s are born twice while the Shudra is born only once. The Shudra is placed outside the accepted social hierarchy in the society and loses the sacred rights, unlike the three twice-born castes. In today’s society, essentially the same Shudras comprises Dalits of today, including a few other social groups.

2.1 Understanding Dalits and Dalit Identity

The term "Dalit" is derived from the Sanskrit root "dal", which means burst, split, crushed, destroyed. Though the term has ancient roots, its contemporary usage to specify a section of the people of India who have suffered oppression throughout history under the prevailing religious and social norms goes back only a few decades. The well-known Hindi dictionary *Bhasa-Shabd-Kosh* describes Dalits as "an undeveloped or backward section of people, such as among the Hindu untouchables (*achut*) or serving caste (*Shudra*)". In Punjabi, however, the *Mahan-Shabd-Kosh* dictionary of Bhai Kahan Singh defines a Dalit as "One who belongs to the lowest caste (*hiniJati*) and has been trampled down by or broken under the feet of the upper caste (*unchijatan*)" (Massey 1997).

The term "Dalits" generally encompasses the communities known as untouchables, Scheduled Castes, and tribes officially treated as Scheduled Tribes (The Bhopal Document 2002).

The ancient root of the term Dalit in Marathi is generally defined as "ground" or "broken to pieces". With the emergence of the "Dalit Panther" movement, the term "Dalit" emerged to have connotations far beyond the simple meaning given above. Eleanor Zelliot illustrates that the underlying implications of the concept of Dalit refers-the people who have been broken, ground down by those above them deliberately and in a playful way. The word in itself has an inherent denial of pollution, Karma, and a justified system of caste hierarchy (cited from The Bhopal Document, 2002).

Through the identity assertion of the Dalits, the word Dalit came to act not only as a definition of a state of degradation and deprivation but also as a significant source of identity and pride. Further, this gave an impetus to use the word "Dalit," the socio-political importance (of which) has increased drastically over the past decade.

The seeds of this understanding lie in the writings of two great Indian personalities, the nineteenth-century reformer and revolutionary Jyotiba Phule, and the twentieth-century intellectual and revolutionary B. R. Ambedkar. In 1973, the Dalit Panthers movement of Maharashtra published its manifesto, "Who is a *Dalit*?" The manifesto answers: "members of Scheduled Castes and Scheduled Tribes, Neo-Buddhist, the working people, the landless and the poor peasants, women and all those who are being exploited politically, economically and in the name of religion" (Massey 1997).

In historical development, many restrictions were imposed on the Shudras. They were prohibited from milking a cow whose milk was to be used in the *Agnihotra*, from taking *Soma* (drink- a drink that produces immortality), from the *upanayana* initiation (or wearing the sacred thread), from studying *Vedas*. The *Vedas* could not even be cited before Dalits or Shudras by law.

The concept of *Varnas* in the context of manual scavengers seems invaluable because they are never considered within the periphery of caste structure, based on *Varna* Vyavastha (Varna system). Dalits, being scavengers, stay at the outskirts of mainstream society. The four *Varnas* based on the hierarchical setup are divided very sharply. The concerned literature suggests, the meaning of *Varnas* is colour, and it was used to define the features of different groups of people, particularly concerning fair Arya with Dark Dasa. The lowest *Varna* was not given a clear and well-defined work to perform, which paved the way to exploitation.

Very briefly, if we study the nomenclature of manual scavengers across the country, it varies irrespectively. As a result, they are known neither as "manual scavengers" nor "sweeper up of dust". The Chuhra is termed "Khakrob". As a domestic servant, he is ironically styled "Mehtar" or "Chieftain", which is an honorific title of various social groups "Bhatiyara," "Qasai". As a worker in the skin or hide, he is called a "Dhed" (literally, "crow") in Gujarat; as a weaver, he is styled "Megh" at least in Rajasthan and, as an executioner, he is known as "Jallad". Further, as a tanner, the Chuhra is called a "Khatik" in Punjab, and as a breeder of swine, he is known as "*Hali*" (Lal, 1999).

2.2 Conceptual Framework

The concept of Dalit is operationalised for this study as follows: "those Scheduled Castes and untouchables who are at present engaged in paid work which is designed as 'polluted' and 'unclean'. These jobs include scavenging, sewerage cleaning, night soil carrying, removing carcasses and dealing with dead bodies at cremations". The following chapters discuss this in detail.

Against the backdrop of the description in the last section, Dalits seem a very special category. This idea will have more significance when the socio-economic conditions of Dalit scavengers are revealed. There has been little work on the communities involved in scavenging, especially on the issues related to their health status. Historically, in every aspect of social life, Dalits and Dalit scavengers have been forced to carry out the most degrading jobs in society. Manual scavenging as an occupation has multiple exploitative phenomena and forms in society. They are the people who generally belong to the lowest strata of Indian society, i.e. of the caste system. They perform the lowest ranking and most degrading jobs in society. The entire urban settlement is based on the continuous cleaning and scavenging taken up by the Hadi community. The neighbouring Bauri caste is not engaged in menial jobs.

A certain kind of occupation is concerned and attached with the operational definition of ***Dalits***. The concepts of pollution and purity, especially, have a clear and direct implication on the lives of Dalits. As there are several theoretical understandings about the origin of caste in India, the emergence of the lower-ranking communities within the caste fold is found in all explanations.

Functional sociologists are concerned with the question of order. This theory believes that every society is a well-integrated structure. Every element as a member of a society has a function that contributes to maintaining the social system. The functioning of the social structure is based on a consensus of its members' values. Exclusively, this school believes that every society is a relatively persistent, stable structure.

The above theory focuses on the functional approach to understanding the caste system, which the dominant Hindu ideology has propagated. **There is always discrimination within the caste system resulting in economic inequality**. It seems necessary to understand the magnitude of caste-based economic inequality in this context. There are three broad theoretical approaches, which attempt to see the economic basis of prevailing institutional consequences of the caste system, the economic efficiency, and income distribution.

Thorat (2001) gives three basic theories in the context of economic efficiency and income distribution:

1. Neo-Classical Approach: This theory assumes that under the prevailing form of the caste system, occupations are hereditary, compulsory, and indigenous. These distinct features of the caste system force immobility in the factors of production, particularly labour, across caste-attached occupations and thus give rise to segmentation in the labour market. The argument is that discrimination exists because of economic incentives.

2. Marxist Approach: This approach focuses on the efficiency aspect of the institution to distribution, as it traces caste-based inequality in the unequal distribution of property. This approach considers the economic structure of the society as the foundation for all the institutions. Focus is given to the dialectical relationship between the changes in the forces of production, i.e. means of production and technology, and the relation of production to the technology. The force of production is supposed to provide a more potent and dynamic source of institutional change. This approach does not feature caste in the arguments relating to the perpetuation of inequality.

3. Ambedkar's Approach: Ambedkar's view on the caste system and untouchability results from the interaction between the Neo-Classical and Marxist theories mentioned above. Ambedkar looked closely at the role and impact of social, religious and philosophical elements in Hinduism in the origin, perpetuation, and sustenance of the caste system. He also analysed the economics of the caste system and untouchability from allocative economic efficiency and income distribution. However, he arrived at a different conclusion. In Ambedkar's view, the Hindu social system involved a framework of a production organisation and a scheme of distribution at a theoretical level.

Hence, different social thinkers have raised the issue of Dalits, but the recent school of Dalits have come up from within the same community as discussed in the study of Thorat (2001). A little clarification is necessary. A few occupational and social groups do not belong to Hinduism. However, they have been carrying out the work and duties of Hindu Dalits because of the importance placed on occupation in the determination of one's life or identity. Many of them have their deities and some practice Buddhism in everyday rituals and rites.

This conceptual understanding is based on the occupation of certain caste groups, which has implications for the health of that same community. The differentiation in health status among different caste groups is found to be because of differences in the socio-economic condition of the respective caste groups.

Similarly, the argument could be applied to the Indian context; the lower socio-economic condition of Dalits and unhygienic environmental living and working conditions means Dalits always have a higher risk of getting exposed to various diseases due to their occupation. No doubt, the health of this section of our population is worse and horrible. Hunger is an important aspect that affects the health of an individual. Rakku's story of Zurbrigg (1984) is a testimony that reflects the live presentation, which reflects the trivial relationship between hunger, health and illness.

The intention behind this study on Dalit health is given in a preliminary sketch to help orientate the readers.

3. Objectives of the Study

3.1. To analyse the socio-economic profile of the Dalit community engaged in "polluted" jobs to locate the overall health conditions and various indicators of the socio-economic condition.

(i) The level of literacy among the Dalits compared with that of the total population is stressed.

(ii) The living and working conditions among Dalits against those of the general population are analysed; other types of work available are stated.

(iii) The total number of the workforce (Dalits) employed, unemployed, or semi-employed is considered in the study.

(iv) The jobs that are viewed to be or considered as "polluted jobs" and the castes involved in these are to be analysed.

3.2. To consider the implications these "polluted jobs" have on the health of this particular community.

(i) How much of the population is adequately housed and the different kinds of housing facilities available.

(ii) How many people still do not have proper food every day.

Accordingly, the traditional occupation of each Dalit caste is being asked and analysed in their current jobs and occupational association.

3.3. To understand or paint a broad picture of the perception about ill health according to the following steps:

(i) The pattern of reported ill-health among this community,

(ii) The utilisation of health care services,

(iii) The socio-physical accessibility to health care services.

4. Area of the Research Study

The place of the study was chosen by enquiring about the caste-based population engaged in the degraded works such as scavenging, cleaning and carrying night soil on their heads etc.

Chas is a township of the district Bokaro in Jharkhand, comprising a total population of 565,290, among which the Scheduled Castes population numbers 66,712. Chas Municipal Corporation has a total Scheduled Caste population of 6,624, and among this, males account for 3,487 and females for 3,137 (Census of India 1991), which has increased to 109,837 in the 2011 census enumeration.

On discovering the above figures of the Chas Municipality, it was decided to undertake a comprehensive survey of the area around the Municipal Corporation. It was found that within this area, Hadi Cooli, a Dalit-populated locality (Cooli refers to a small settlement Dalits), is engaged in scavenging, cleaning latrines and carrying night soil etc. So the Hadi Cooli was selected for the research study, which consisted of only forty-eight households in the year 2001, all of them from the same occupation.

Mehtar has a significant space in this area of exploitation. *Hadi,* a sub-caste of Mehtar, is found in the Chas Township of Bokaro district. People from both of these castes preach Hinduism.

5. Methods of Data Collection

Primary and secondary have been used to attain the overall proposed study objectives. Earlier only forty-eight households settled in Hadi Cooli were selected because of their rugged, congested housing conditions and the surrounding environment.

5.1 Tools

5.1.1 Interview schedule: The interview schedule was applied to gather factual and quantitative data from the respondents. Out of the total 48 households, 36 were interviewed. Interviews were supplemented and helped by a prepared checklist to guide and facilitate the interview schedule and discussion with the respondents.

5.1.2 In-depth interview: In-depth interviews were carried out with selected respondents to increase the reliability and quality of the field data.

5.1.3 Focus Group Discussions (FGDs): This technique had some difficulty; gathering community fellows in one place at one time was extremely difficult. FGDs were done with other Dalit communities, who live near the Hadi Cooli area, known as (the) Bauri Cooli (Bauri is a caste that belongs to the Scheduled Caste but is not involved in scavenging). This was helpful to relate the issues to broader socio-economic factors.

5.1.4 Case Study

The case study method helped bring hidden aspects of Dalit's life to light. For this purpose, five individuals were selected who had significance in manifesting a higher mortality rate of those in their families. This method revealed the factors responsible for their lower health status.

The data collected was related to their living conditions, healthcare-seeking behaviour, availability and accessibility of health services, the reasons for non-accessibility, the diseases prominently occurring in the settlement area, their employment, nutrition, and housing problems.

6. Scope and Limitation of the Study

The study area was not significant regarding the number of settled households. Out of forty-eight, only thirty-eight (38) respondents were interviewed because the rest could not be found even after many visits, and a few did not want to talk. Most of the time, especially in the early morning and evening hours, they were not available at home because of their busy work hours. To catch the men at home, the researcher had to inform them one day in advance, but the women were available most of the time except when they would go out to collect drinking water from the public tap.

The tools and techniques of data collection applied, such as In-depth Interviews and Focus Group Discussions, were the most effective methods for collecting qualitative data. However, these methods demand a long time and energy for the intensive and comprehensive study.

Another thing that needs to be mentioned here that may have affected the study was the relationship with the community. In the first few days, the researcher had to enter the community with the assistance of the Registered Medical Practitioner (RMPs) and a few other local interactive and vocal community members. However, later the researcher succeeded in building up his rapport with the community. However, a non-participant observation method was used as a supplementary instrument throughout the research study.

7. Scheme of the Chapter plan

This book is based on a study done in the Chas Township, a part of the Bokaro district in the newly formed state of Jharkhand. It is about a community of Dalits engaged mainly in the occupation of scavenging who carry the night soil and clean the toilets of the thousands of houses in Bokaro city, located on the banks of river Garga. The city is the site of a large government-owned steel plant, which started its production in 1978. After failing to gain financial and technical aid from the United States to construct the steel plant, in 1965, the Indian government reached an agreement with the Union of Soviet Socialist Republics (USSR), which provided the necessary support. A major rail line and a national highway link Bokaro to other cities. The nearest domestic airport is Patna, about 225 kilometres to the northwest, in Bihar state.

The research study is based on primary data collected in the field and secondary sources such as various government documents, books, journals and magazines, newspaper clippings, etc.

The first chapter deals with the study's rationale and its conceptual framework. It also gives an idea about the hypothesis prepared to go into the field, the research methodology adopted for data collection, and the sociology of health and social exclusion.

The second chapter comprises socio-historical accounts of Dalits' particular reference to Hadis. The third chapter provides a socio-demographic and economic profile, and the fourth chapter describes the socio-demographic profile of the study area and explores Dalits' health. The fifth chapter, "The Axes of Denial", explains the data on the perception and reported morbidity among the selected study population and the links between health and social exclusion of *Hadis*. The final chapter discusses practices, findings and conclusions based on observations of the research.

CHAPTER TWO

SOCIO-HISTORICAL ACCOUNTS OF DALITS WITH SPECIAL REFERENCE TO HADI CASTE

1. Introduction

The word "*Dalit*" in itself has been a matter of extensive debate. The usage of Dalit got its genesis in Marathi literature as discussed in the earlier chapter. Similar to how every society has some form of social and literary explanation for particular activities and incidents occurring in that society, the structural differences are rooted in historicity of the society and culture as caste has its root in the ancient scriptures of Hinduism. Quite specifically, the historicity of the term "Dalit" is rooted in the struggles of Dalit movements in western India and later expanded across the Indian states playing a crucial role in the writings upon Dalit life and community. The concept of *Dalit* has now turned out to be a fashionable issue to look into but the important aspect of this argument is how much it is relevant to discuss. Do we mean that Dalits are found only among the Hindu caste system or also in others? If yes, then, how is the role of religion defined in determining the social status of *Dalits* irrespective of religious communities?

A major factor in the life of a Dalit is to only ever be a Dalit for the rest of his/her life. There have been several attempts to breakdown the barrier of caste, citing the reason that change in the Hindu social structure that governs the life of people in the society, is little flexible but caste structure is rigid as it has bases from Hindu religious scriptures. The conversion movements were led by Dr. B.R. Ambedkar in 1956 and later a few Ambedkarites also attempted to choose similar path to get rid from the burden of caste atrocities and inequality, the case of Udit Raj was one. The caste system is too deeply embedded in the daily life of Indians and the social, economic, and political sphere: it can be observed in every single activity of an individual in India. A large number of low caste-born families are located at the margins of the society and the same group got called Dalits initially in western India. It was

Dalit Panther movements that asserted the identity of low caste born people and give them a commonly known name 'Dalit'. Dalits are, no doubt, exploited groups but the difference varies within the Dalits as to the differences in their religion.

The history of untouchability also varies according to different sources. Theological sources of history talk differently compared to other sources. The evidence regarding the genesis of caste also varies from region to region. The conflicts between Aryan and Dravidian scholars are based on their logic and reasons. Aryans as invaders had a common religion and language that were highly self-aware made the upper caste Hindus as the powerful group in India, though historically they were outsiders to India. They began their invasions of India from the north-west around 1500 B.C. Hutton's idea, in *Caste in India: Its nature, functions, and origin* (1963) was to briefly illustrate the origin of caste and division of labour before Aryan tribes in India and how they made efforts at self-preservation in the face of further invasions.

There is a widespread belief that caste and caste-based untouchability can be traced back to the Aryans and how they positioned themselves at their initial encounter with India's indigenous populace. For ages, Aryans have been thought to have had recurring confrontations with the people of the Indian subcontinent. The belief was that Aryans looked down on indigenous people as inferior and feeble, excluding them from all rites and declaring them unclean. In post-Rig Vedic literature, there are several references to primitive woodland inhabitants held on the periphery of Aryan culture in conquered areas. They were named the Chandal (Webster, 1994).

Untouchability appears to have taken root between 600B.C. and 200 A.D. (Webster 1994) when it became a stigma attached to a particular group of people. The Chandalas were severely stigmatised in the later Vedic Age, and references to social rank became important. The "mixed caste theory" of the origins of untouchability started on the basis of the descriptions given in the Dharmasutras and in Kautilya's famous book *Arthasastra*, where the Chandala are treated as untouchable. The classic explanation of the Varna system theory and the differentiation based on occupational hierarchy in the form of castes related to "pollution" was given only in the Manusmriti (ibid.). The classification of castes according to the four Varnas is the dominant theoretical explanation (Gupta 1991). Brahmins, Kshatriyas, Vaishyas, and Shudras (Jhunjhunwala 1999), all created by the Lord Brahma. Each group consists of different castes and is restricted in terms of food, marriage, rituals, and festivals and so on. Varna represents the system of values, whereas castes represent the occupational organisation. Caste was supposed to represent a social organisation to assist all individuals in fulfilling their desires in a socially harmonious way (ibid.). Each caste has different sub-castes based on endogamous groups. Caste can be studied as a unit to study the Indian society and associated outcomes in the form of discrimination and unequal system that it brought and made functional as a unit caste is identified by the birth of an individual in a specific family, whereas as a system, caste is represented as an interrelated status and through the pattern of interaction between different castes relating to different prohibitions.

However, it is also argued that Manu did not come up with the idea of caste and that caste actually existed long before Manu. Manu was an upholder of it and therefore [1] philosophised in such a way that it inherently turned out to be a common part of common belief not only as a concept of caste but as an everyday practice. His work ended with the codification of existing caste rules and preaching of caste Dharma (WSBRA 1979).

2. Sociological Politics of Census

It is pertinent to study the caste census and its implications on the kind of studies and research that follows from it in the social sciences domain. The enumeration of *Dalits* as a Scheduled Castes in the [1] Census of India (2001) immensely helps to understand the pragmatic aspects of most disadvantaged communities in India, especially the social groups engaged in impure and "polluted" occupations. The sociological politics in the Census is important to analyse the occupational categorisation of castes groups in India. The purpose of the Census was primarily social engineering to facilitate the British Empire in India than uncover the social structure of the Indian population. Michael Mann, in his book *South Asia's Modern History: Thematic Perspectives* (2015), writes that the census exercise was "more telling the administrative needs of the British than of the social reality for the people of British India" (2015: 169). The sociological implications of the data collection on 'caste', 'religion', occupation, and age and so on had a considerable impact on the socio-political agenda of the society. M. N. Srinivas (1942) observed in his long anthropological study in a village of Mysore that people began changing their caste groups in order to attain better social status and, therefore, reported to the census enumerator in their region to correct their caste names and surnames.

2.1 The Politico-Administrative Context of Caste in India

There are twenty-three Scheduled Castes listed in the special issue of Scheduled Castes (SCs) and Scheduled Tribes (STs) in the 1971 Census of India reports. They are; Bantar, Bauri, Bhogta, Bhuiya, Bhumij (excluding North Chhotanagpur & South Chhotanagpur division and Santhal Pragana district), Chamar/Mochi, Dabgar, Dholi, Dom and Dhangad, Dusadh- Dhari and Dharhi, Ghasi, Halalkhor, Hari-Mehtar and Bhangi, Kenjar, Kuraniar, Lalbegi, Musahar, Nat, Pan and Sawari, Pasi, Rajwar, Turi (Census of India 1971).

Among the above 23 castes, most are engaged in different jobs usually considered menial in the social hierarchy and occupational structure. These castes in Indian society are defined as "polluted" and menial. Mehtar and Bhangis are the common caste groups engaged in carrying night soil. However, this is not strictly defined because Lalbegi and Halalkhor are also engaged in the same work (Lal 1999).

The first Census of India was undertaken in 1881 (WSBRA), during the period of colonial empire when no Indian voices could be heard raised before the ruler. Since the mutiny of 1857, the country's state of affairs had been in the hands of the British. The British had never lost any opportunities to govern India on the "divide and rule" policy, and the introduction of caste in the census only consolidated the British rule in India more systematically. However, according to B.R. Ambedkar, "it was a bold and good step to know the real number of the castes and creed that existed. It seems ridiculous because we did not bother about the classes that did not favour this initiation. It helped to know and calculate the total population in the Census of India (colonial) in 1881. The first attempt to classify Hindus based on caste, race and grade in the Census of 1881 was crude. The steps towards an organized classification were made with the initiative of census enumeration" (WSBRA 1989).

The next Census of India taken in 1901 was based on a new approach to classify the population "by social precedence as recognised by native public opinion" (ibid., 6). But this approach faced an organised resistance from the upper castes of the Hindus. As regards the numerical strength of the Dalits, or untouchables, there has been a vast vacuum in counting the total Dalit population. The "Census of 1911 laid down ten tests to mark off the untouchables and it was the beginning of the ascertainment of the population of untouchables. Efforts continued in the same direction in the Census of 1921 and 1931. The Simon commission gave the figure of untouchables in British India as 44.5 million" (ibid.7). The Hindu upper *Varna* caste, especially Brahmins, have always protested against the separate census of untouchables. This tendency is still prevalent today and serious opposition emerged by different sections on this issue in the enumeration process by caste in the Census report of 2001. The resistance did not sway the present census commissioner, who is of the view that census enumeration by caste is very important. Establishing the importance of considering caste for any viable discussion on India's population. Regardless of one's feelings about caste as a social structure, Ambedkar asserted that "it is hard to think of any useful discussion of population issues in India without caste being a significant part" and that "caste is still the foundation of the Indian social fabric." The caste system continues to be the best predictor of changes in India's various social policies (WSBRA 1979). Ambedkar thought that every Hindu is born into a caste and that his caste shapes his entire life, including his religious, social, economic, and personal life.

The crucial steps to identify the difference and distinctions between castes were taken in 1911 through the Census of India, which laid down ten tests to mark out the untouchables from those who were touchable. The Census superintendent made a "separate enumeration of castes and tribes who (1) denied the supremacy of the Brahmin or other recognised Hindu Guru, (3) denied the authority of the *Vedas*, (4) did not worship the great Hindu Gods; (5) were not served by good Brahmins, (6) had no Brahmin priests at all; (7) had no access to the interior of an ordinary Hindu temple; (8) caused pollution; (9) bury their dead and (10) eat beef and did not reverence the cow" (ibid., 19). The high caste Hindu population rejected this because it seemed dangerous to them. However, the figures of 1951 were published and widely debated.

The point is to assess the health scenario of scavengers. According to the 1961 Census of India, only 48.2 per cent of the total number of persons engaged in sweeping, scavenging and allied occupations belonged to the Scheduled Castes category. Major scavenging castes in the eastern part of India are Hari-Mehtar, mainly found in carrying night soil on their heads or in baskets.

As a result, Dalits' social conditions have deteriorated to the point of oppression, aggravating their already precarious living conditions. Here, health is a critical factor that must be considered. Untouchability based on caste has been a unique phenomenon in India: a hereditary order in rank and function.

When you are Touchable, you are always Touchable. If you've ever been untouchable, you will always be untouchable. When you're a Brahmin, you're a Brahmin for life. When you're a sweeper, you're always a sweeper. Those who are born high stay high, and those who are born low stay low. In another way, the established order is based on a certain law of Karma that is set in stone once and for all. This fate has nothing to do with the merits of the people who live under it (WSBRA, 1989). Isn't it a dilemma in a society established based on caste hierarchy, with a background of a subsidised economy under foreign domination and uneven distribution of modern education? While India's constitution pledges to create a democratic and egalitarian society (Prasad, 1990).

The debate on caste and untouchability is relevant to understanding Dalit issues in general and scavengers in particular. The question of untouchability was raised in the Durban conference held between the third of August and the seventh of September 2001. The agreement there was that, like race, caste is based on the United Nations definition of "colour (*Varna*), descent and ethos" fortified by many years of the strictest rules of endogamy, social segregation, pollution and subjugation by the upper caste Brahmins who were canonized by divine interdictions to preserve purity of blood and ethnic superiority" (Dalit Voice, 2001).

2.2. Dalits in the field of Literature and Writing

The ancient writers Valmiki, Vyasa, and Kalidasa, were not Brahmins, but they all came from impoverished backgrounds. Satyakama Jabala, a vital philosopher who wrote the Sanskrit book Aranyakas, too hailed from a low social class. It demonstrates that Brahmins were not the only ones who spoke Sanskrit. Those who excelled in philosophy and literature were treated as Brahmins and were considered honourable members of the learned.

However, the duality within the history of Indian classes is significant because one may argue both ways by citing other examples of caste-based organisations. Eklavya was denied education learned archery, but he was not twice-born and had a meagre school budget. Ancient Hindu civilisation is not amenable to broad generalisations" (Nadkarni 1997).

Even so, after the days of Eklavya, Hindu civilisation did not remain stagnant. Gautam Buddha is thought to have been the first to condemn the caste system and reject the scriptures that justified it. This step was taken before the Bhakti movement, which rejected the Brahminic language

'Sanskrit' and taught their doctrine in people's native languages" after a lengthy period of silence (ibid.).

2.3 The Scavengers: an Exploited Class

The scavengers or sweepers have many synonyms in different parts of the country. As a scavenger or rather a "sweeper up of dust," the *Chuhra* is termed *Khakrob,* like "Dalits". If we look at the Dalits in undivided Bihar, the 1981 Census of India (for SC/ST tables of Bihar) has mentioned twenty-three Scheduled Castes. However, only a few of them are still found engaged in "polluted jobs" under the category of "main workers seeking 'special occupation' in the Census classification on workers" (Census of India, 1971). In this category, three sub-categories are identified as follows:

(1) Seeking / available for work.
(2) Scavenging.
(3) Tanning and currying of hides and skins.

The seriously miserable condition of Dalits is that they do not have a recorded history: A mass of 250 million outcastes comprising the untouchables and the tribes are grappling with history and survival at the turn of the millennium. They have always been outside the *Varna* system. The untouchables remained a part of the village economy but were segregated to remain outside the village and perform menial services. Untouchables, over time, were denied civil rights, including the right to possess wealth, acquire knowledge, and possess arms. Tribals pushed away into infertile areas and were geographically segregated. All through the (history) centuries, Dalits have suffered the most barbaric forms of oppression unparalleled in world history (The Bhopal Document, 2002).

Susan Chaplin (1997) gives different accounts of the failure of governmental initiatives. Scavengers are still carrying nightsoil, including the sanitary services in cities and towns. Excluding a small number who are engaged with different municipal or local urban authorities, a large number of them are still engaged in their traditional occupation. There is no doubt that scavenger's still carry nightsoil in baskets on their heads, as their work has always been polluted according to Hindu society. Hence scavengers are treated as untouchable, even by other untouchable castes". The question of the opportunities available to Dalits, especially scavengers, has great importance. The simple explanation is that since scavengers are polluted, whatever they do or touch will become polluted. Chaplin rightly says that discrimination refers to the scavengers having few or limited job opportunities other than sanitary work. They live in acute poverty in segregated communities and have extremely low literacy and job mobility levels. Such a pathetic socio-economic condition of scavengers persist despite the various provisions and protective articles in the constitution of India, which instruct the state to promote the economic and educational interests of Scheduled Castes and protect them from discrimination and exploitation. We will now look at the measures taken to protect Dalits' rights after adopting the Indian constitution on 26th November (1949).

3. Constitutional Measures

The constitution of India takes serious note of the existing problem regarding untouchability. There are many provisions under various articles, 15 (2), 17, 29 (2), which consider the practice of untouchability as an offence (Shah, 2001). Many people view that the most significant movement initiated by any person was no other than Mahatma Gandhi. Gandhi dedicated his life to freeing manual scavengers from the painful and dishonourable task of manually cleaning human excrement and grime.

Mahatma Gandhi was criticised mainly for all he did for the upliftment of scavengers. He said, "I do not want to attain Moksha; I do not want to be reborn. However, suppose I have to be reborn. In that case, I should be born an untouchable so that I may share their sorrows, sufferings, and the efforts levelled at them to endeavour to free myself and them from that miserable condition. I, therefore, pray that should I be born again that I should do so not as a Brahmin, Kshatriya, Vaishya or Shudra but as an Atisudra, a Bhangi" (Srivastava, 1997: 35).

This ideology and aspiration were practised in the Gandhi Ashram, and scavenging was carried out by the Ashramites irrespective of caste and dignity. Shah writes that atrocities against Dalits have not gone down recently. He gives an example of the new Scheduled Castes and Scheduled Tribes (Prevention of Atrocities Act, 1989) promulgated in Gujarat (Shah 2001).

3.1 Recommendations of Various Committees/Commissions

3.1.1 Barve committee

Scavenging has been an omnipresent occupation found in most states and state premises. The Barve committee was entrusted to suggest best ways and sustainable means to improve working conditions and fix a minimum wage for scavengers. The committee submitted the report to the Government of Bombay in 1952. The Ministry of Home Affairs articulated a copy of the major recommendations to all the state governments and requested them adopt those recommendations. The recommendations were widely capable of optimum application and could have been implemented profitably. The Ministry of Health took another action plan, Government of India to address the conditions of manual scavengers (Srivastava, 1997) showing initiative to address the concerns of manual scavengers at ministerial levels.

3.1.2 Scheme for the supply of wheelbarrows

The Government of India suggested supplying wheelbarrows/ handcarts to sweepers employed by municipalities for scavenging work. This initiative was an initial step to make scavenging more consistent with human dignity and respect to work. The intention to eradicate carrying nightsoil as head load could be abolished. To facilitate this implementation, the government of India provided fifty per cent of the actual costs towards the purchase of wheelbarrows/ handcarts through the state governments. The response from the different local bodies was not considerable and this did not work properly. It was reported that the wheelbarrows provided were mostly improper, quite heavy to carry. Manual scavengers found it more convenient to discard the tools than to face problems while using it (Srivastava, 1997). At present, a lot has changed due to continuous pressure and re-thinking how to handle manual scavengers in India and how to get these works done mechanically.

3.1.3 Kaka Kalelkar Commission

The first report of the Backward Classes Commission, set up by a presidential order on 29th January 1953 adhering to Article 340 of the Constitution of India, under the chairmanship of Kaka Kalelkar, was submitted in 1955. The commission observed that the working and living condition of sweepers and scavengers were inhuman. Bhangis clean latrines/toilets to maintain health and sanitation in society at the cost of the risk to their health and life. The entire population would have to face nearly epidemics, had they not been doing this filthiest job. In addition to this, they are forced to live in the filthiest surroundings. It is common sight observing them carrying nightsoil on their heads in the old city and town where Municipalities have not been available to clean with the help of tools and they cannot give excuses like lack of resources. Unfortunately the fate of this recommendation was the same as that of others. At least, the Ministry of Home Affairs shared and brought these observations and recommendations to the notice of all the state governments in October, 1956. Ministry emphasized the need to introduce mechanical and most advanced cleaning methods. It intended to minimize this inhuman practice of manual cleaning and carrying nightsoil as head loads (Srivastava, 1997).

3.1.4 Central Advisory Board for Harijan Welfare

A year after submitting the Kalelkar Commission report, the Ministry of Home Affairs constituted another committee known as Central Advisory Board of Harijan Welfare in 1956. This board was under the chairmanship of the late Pandit Gobind Ballabh Pant. It was observed in the board's report that the working and living conditions of the sweepers and manual scavengers in the country are disgraceful and inhuman. They recommended to the Government of India to bring a centrally sponsored scheme to eradicate the practice of scavenging (ibid., 37-38).

3.1.5 Malkani Committee

Under the chairmanship of N. R. Malkani and four other members, this committee argued for putting "an end to the degrading practice of scavenging and carrying nightsoil in buckets or baskets. It recommended not merely for eliminating the practice of carrying night soil as head loads. This committee also recommended for bringing faith and dignity in all life stages of scavenging and for improving the working and living conditions and social status of the community" (ibid., 38).

3.1.6 Committee on Customary Rights to Scavenging

In 1965, the Central Department of Social Welfare established the Committee on Customary Rights to Scavenging. In modern and independent India, this governmental committee had a considerable impact on identifying social groups suffering from backwardness and excessive cruel treatment.

3.1.7 Pandya Committee (The National Commission on Labour constituted by the Union Ministry of Labour appointed sub-committee)

Another attempt to address the concerns of scavenging communities was the Pandya Committee. During 1967-68, India's government created a sub-committee on Sweepers and Scavengers under the Union Ministry of Labour. It was suggested that the working and living conditions of sweepers and scavengers be investigated, as they were not improving despite previous attempts. There were a few similar state-level committees that attempted to address the cessation of manual scavenging, including Uttar Pradesh (1955), Haryana (1969), Kerala (1971), and Karnataka (1976).

3.1.8 Improvement in the working and living conditions of those engaged in unclean occupations

During the Third Five-Year Plan (1961–1966), the Ministry of Home Affairs of the Government of India implemented a centrally supported and sponsored scheme in response to the Malkani Committee's several recommendations. It is divided into two parts: (i) bettering the working conditions of sweepers, scavengers, tenors, and flyers, and (ii) bettering the living situations of Scheduled Castes who worked in unsanitary occupations or were landless labourers. The project, however, failed and was phased down during the fifth five-year plan.

3.1.9 Gandhi Centenary Year

On the occasion of Gandhi Centenary Year in 1969, the Government of India launched a revolutionary programme to convert dry latrines into water-pour flush latrines, a novel technique to remove the practice of scavenging. A 25% subsidy to households was granted under this system, with the remaining 75% as a repayable loan in instalments.

Several committees have made proposals in response to the dreadful and deplorable state of scavengers' lives and their surroundings. In the worst-case scenario, most of the committees' recommendations had little long-term influence and failed to meet their objectives. Throughout policy and implementation, there has been a lack of devotion and apathy for the cause of sweeping and manual scavenging, according to objective analysis. The state's concern has just been identified.

The role of non-governmental organisations has excellent potential to stop manual scavenging. The Sulabh International Social Service Organisation (2001), for example, started quite early and has been carrying out practical work in this direction to liberate scavengers. However, Sulabh's initiative does criticise how the organisation employs people from low-caste groups in its all-Indian toilet chain. Furthermore, why does Sulabh employs only manual scavenging castes members in the chain of public toilets across the country? So why not another caste? It needs another study to examine this perspective. A few prominent voluntary organisations are involved in the cause of liberating scavengers; they are the Harijan Sevak Sangh and Safai

Vidyalaya, Ahmedabad; Safai Karamchari Andolan, Navsirjan and Gandhi Smark Nidhi, Pune.

Non-governmental organisations can play an essential role in ending manual scavenging. For example, the Sulabh International Social Service Organization (2001) started early and has been doing practical work to free scavengers ever since. Sulabh's effort, on the other hand, has been criticised for employing people from low caste groups in its toilet network across India. Furthermore, why does Sulabh employ members of the manual scavenging castes in its nationwide network of public toilets solely? So why not add another caste to the mix? Another study is required to investigate this viewpoint. The Harijan Sevak Sangh and Safai Vidyalaya in Ahmedabad, the Safai Karamchari Andolan in Navsirjan, and Gandhi Smark Nidhi in Pune are among the significant voluntary organisations working to free scavengers.

4. Dalits and Atrocities

The concept of untouchability has waned in theory and in practice, and its flaws have been widely explored since India's independence. However, the number of events involving Dalits has increased, not reduced. They are mostly disregarded, and the crimes committed against Dalits include murder, grievous bodily harm, fire, and rape, among other things. According to Kamble (1992), the following crimes occurred in the following order:

1. Firing the house of Dalit families after locking them inside.
2. To burn alive.
3. Brutal murdering of untouchables.
4. Risking or sacrificing the life in the pretext of rituals and sacrifice.
5. Beating and stripping women naked through the village and beating or raping them in broad daylight.
6. Prohibition to fetch drinking water from common wells and making filthy by pouring excreta into Dalit's drinking water wells or throwing dead carcases of animals etc.
7. Damaging the grown-up crops in their farms and lands.
8. Forcing Dalits to follow tradition is harmful to their dignity and interests, as it prevents them from expressing their rights as citizens in all aspects of society, including the right to join temples.

The cruel nature of social reality is fiercely damaging the life of any Dalit in society. Scavengers are harshly treated and have never abandoned the traditional occupation that humiliates them daily.

Susan Chaplin (1997) writes that scavengers are politically relatively weak, adding vulnerability. He provides an account of the atrocities meted out to scavengers in the following:

(1) Scavengers cannot apply political pressure on the state/government to ensure their living and working conditions.
(2) They lack effective political representation and influence because they are a minority group among Scheduled Castes (SCs).
(3) There is a slight possibility of scavengers establishing political alliances because of their isolation from other low caste groups.
(4) Scavenging remains a complex socioeconomic and cultural issue. This Hindu caste-based social order burden necessitates proper and optimal resourcing and the will of both the state and society. In order to alleviate this customary load, Indian culture must undergo a fundamental shift in mindset.

These facts cannot be thrown aside/ignored because the levels of atrocities suffered/experienced by Dalits and also by scavengers have only continued to rise/increase in numbers but not minimized. As previously stated, Dalits are found in India and a few other nations in South Asia, including Nepal, Bangladesh, Sri Lanka, and Pakistan. Bosco (2001) describes how encouraging scavenging has influenced the Indian Diaspora in Burma, Malaysia, South Africa, East Africa, the Caribbean, the United Kingdom, Canada, and the United States. He also claims that the Buraku people of Japan, the Osun people of Nigeria, and the Somalian Mitgan are just a few examples of today's so-called egalitarian civilizations rife with injustices and prejudice. The Osu are a Nigerian lower-caste people who are 90% Christians, yet no bishop has been honoured among them so far. Madhiban, also known as the Gaboye, are a Somali artisanal caste. Mitgans in Somalia are low caste, considered impure, unclean, and thus untouchable. These outcastes are not allowed to organize themselves. A famous proverb goes as 'The world will end when the noble caste starts drinking and the Mitgans start praying' (Bosco 2001).

One can see structures similar to the caste system in other parts of the globe; however, the denial of social discrimination and exclusion meted out towards certain social groups in the Hindu caste system is unkind than in others. There is no recognition of individual intellect and potential to perform in the caste society. The knowledge and skills are believed to be ascribed by birth but not learning and personal capability.

Another important aspect is the Scheduled Caste status provided to the castes having faced discrimination and those placed low in the social hierarchy. According to the Constitution (Scheduled Castes), Order, 1950, as amended from time to time, "no person who professes a religion different from the Hindu, the Sikh or Buddhist religion shall be deprived to be a member of a scheduled caste". Srivastava illustrates that not all manual scavengers need to be SCs as per the provision of the Constitution Order, 1950. However, a few scavenging communities are left out from this particular provision. Therefore, it means that a person professing religion other than Hinduism, Sikhism or Buddhism like Christianity, Islam, or tribal cannot be Scheduled Caste (Srivastava, 1997: 19).

The name 'Mehtar' was commonly applied to the servants of the emperor Humayun. Another name for them was "Halalkor": "one who eats what is lawful, one whose earnings are legitimate". There is a famous saying about the origin of a Muslim caste scavenger: "During the reign of Aurangzeb, a corpse was found lying in the streets of Delhi. It appeared to Muslims to be a Hindu corpse and Hindus to be a Muslim one. The Lalbegis were at last ordered to remove it, but as they went to carry it away, it became converted into a heap of flowers" (ibid.: 21).

The Lalbegis claimed this to be "their *Pir Lalbeg* who had come to help them out of their degraded position; the emperor was so struck with the wonder at the change that he allowed the Lalbegis to live in towns and villages and to carry on their profession by day as well as night" (ibid. 21-22). Lalbegis are a low caste born population in India.

In reality scavengers in India are people stigmatised by and from birth and ascribed group membership. Srinivas (1969) describes the characteristics of caste identity as:

1. Hierarchy (being born into a particular caste and maintaining a separate identity through use of caste names).
2. Endogamy and hypergamy (marriage within the caste and outside respectively).
3. Occupational association (caste is identified with a particular profession / occupation).
4. Restriction on food, drink and smoking.
5. Distinction in custom, dress and speech.

6. Pollution (by sight or touch).
7. Ritual and other privileges and disabilities.
8. Caste organisation (caste council and Panchayats etc.).
9. Caste mobility (Caste habitations).

Srivastava (1997) touches very briefly on the idea that the quintessence of caste is written off as by the existence of hereditary groups in a hierarchy. The Brahmin are at the top and Dalit at the bottom where the bottom has always been forced to perform unclean, filthy and impure occupations.

4.1 Dalits and Occupation

While a substantive amount of work on Dalits concentrates on their political participation, *Dalit* identity and occupation, very little are written on their health. Both Dalit and non-Dalit scholars have tried to focus on Dalits as a problem of identity within the framework of the caste system only.

Ravindran (1996) focused on the health of Dalit children, and the data on the mortality and morbidity of this community is either scant or not available. Indian sociological studies tend to cover a broader perspective on Dalits and the social stigma. However, the stigmatisation of a group leads towards the worsening health and sickness of that group is not covered.

There are legal provisions in place to stop the manual carrying and cleaning of night soils: "The Parliament in the Budget session of 1993 passed the 'Employment of manual scavengers and construction of dry latrines (Prohibition) Bill, 1993' to abolish scavenging. It was to ban the construction of dry latrines and engage in or employ for or permit to be engaged in or employed for any other person for manually carrying human excreta." This act has no time limitation for implementation. However, several states, namely Andhra Pradesh, Goa, Karnataka, Maharashtra, Tripura, West Bengal, Bihar and Delhi, have followed the law in their land (Srivastava 1997).

Dalits are primarily at the lowest socioeconomic level, and the poor condition compels them to live in filthy settlements and urban areas in the congested slums. Ahmad (1999) examines the classification of castes based on their occupation and the caste-class nexus as follows.

Classical *Varna* Model Based on Division of Labour

Varna	**Class**	**Deity worshipped**
1. Brahman	Priests, Interpreters of Dharma	Agni
2. Kshatriya	Warriors, Rulers	Indra
3. Vaishya	Commoners, Cattle herders	Visvedeva
4. Shudra	Peasants, workers, servants	

Note: Rigveda mentioned only the first three *Varna*s, Shudra was a later addition.

This model briefs with a message of uncertainty about Dalits, categorised in the last *Varna*s without any proper specification. The question of 'social status', at least apparently, has been central to "untouchables". Their economic status and political power remain substantive factors in determining their position in Indian society (Sharma 1997). According to Dumont (1972), purity-impurity stands on the principle of scalar yardstick, and the fact emerges that a caste is kept different from another caste.

4.2 The Dalit Movement

The Dalit identity-based movement has reduced the speed of Sanskritization at one point. For example, the post-independence period is characterised as converting to Buddhism, primarily when Dr B R Ambedkar converted. This was not an attempt for individual salvation but rather a quest for collective emancipation (Shah 1990). Reform movements among and for Dalits have not yet managed to satisfy Dalit demands. Ghanshyam Shah has classified the Dalit movement into reformative and alternative. A reformative movement focuses on studying changes in the caste system and institution of untouchability.

In contrast, matters relating to conversion to other religions (for example, Buddhism, Islam, Christianity), education, economic status and political power are taken up in the study of alternative movements". When caste becomes politically influential and political parties' electoral campaigns are formed on the liking of caste, there is a higher chance of suppression of the lower class of a caste. One has to be part of a particular caste to run an election.

Dominant communities are seen even among Dalits, like in other caste groups. The history of India shows diversity in the dominance, which has been caste-based. The large number of people participating in the struggle for independence also diversified the nature of the dominant caste group. That is to say, and this group is now more in number, educationally advanced and politically aware. The Kalelkar commission (1955) noted that the Mahars dominate the untouchables in Maharashtra. In northern India, the Chamars are the dominant caste, whereas down in the south, the Ezhavas and Nayars are the dominant community among the other Scheduled Caste groups.

The interaction and participation in political movements started in the pre-independence period inspired the lower caste to start the non-Brahmin movement headed by some leaders of the Maratha community, like the Raja of Kolhapur. This movement was to some extent anti-congress and pro-British and got full support from many Muslims, Christians and others. This movement gained the same support in the southern states of India (Shah 1990).

4.3 Health Concerns

According to the Kaka Kalelkar Commission (1955), health is one of the most important factors of national success in any subject. Nothing is more important than the people's health in a country, which is assessed in terms of their energy and capacity and the potential of person-hours for productive labour concerning the total number of people maintained by the country. Workers' health is a critical factor for any egalitarian society and nation regarding resources for economic development and industry and agriculture efficiency. In terms of resources for economic development and efficiency of industry and agriculture, the worker's health is an essential consideration for any equitable society and a nation.

The majority of marginalised among the lower castes and Dalits are still engaged in scavenging. Seasonal epidemics cause higher mortality among Dalit scavengers, and others will usually suffer from dysentery, malaria and/or tuberculosis. The focus of five plans has been contagious diseases, and Public Health was consolidated as an essential issue for the marginalised.

The Kalelkar Commission noted the need to supply "pure drinking water and stated that public wells and reservoirs must be built within easy reach of the Harijan quarters to use the whole area. They should be maintained in sanitary condition under the supervision of a Village Water Committee (VWC) with Harijan presidents" (ibid., 99).

Two opposite approaches to improving Dalit living conditions have always been discussed. The most dominant voice has been Mahatma Gandhi, who put forward a reformist approach. The basic paradigm of this school is that the problem of evil of the caste system can be reformed while staying within the caste framework and not by changing the whole structure of the caste system. This idea was propagated by most of the Indian functionalist sociologists who resisted the idea of religious conversion. The notion of caste and caste-based purity/pollution determines an individual identity, which is not scientific. People cannot show their worthiness in the overall aspect of livelihood and survival if they are not given the opportunities. By socialisation, the different institutions of Indian society force every caste group and its members to internalise the idea of caste hierarchy and its ritual performance. This is helped by textbooks, undoubtedly and by enforcing the so-called "Brahminical ethos of life".

Ilaiah (1996), through the experiences of everyday life, has critiqued the Hindutva Ideology. He identified the distinctions in the way of life and of a Shudra. This work refers to how children's experiences of growing up as a member of a particular caste, with references to marriage, market and social relations and from trajectories of birth to death of a person either belonging to an upper caste or lower Dalit family.

Ambedkar further strengthened the views of contrasting functionalist sociologists. He questioned the Hindu view of life based on a harmonious pursuit of the four chief conceivable objects of life, viz., Dharma, Artha, Kama and Moksha, but he rejected it by embracing Buddhism and the conversion of Dalits from Hinduism to Buddhism. The same converted group emerged out as Neo-Buddhist. The idea that Hinduism is a religion of humanity is entirely rejected by the followers of Ambedkar and later by the Dalit Panther Movement in the nineteen seventies of the post-independence decades (Shah 2001). Das (2001), while reviewing the work of Kancha Illaiah, stated that the call by Hindu leaders in recent years to promote the Hindutva ideology had raised apprehensions and anxiety among the people of the lower section of society. The rightWing Hindu organisation wishes to continue strengthening the hold of the dominating upper castes upon the Dalits. Illaiah's books *Why I am Not a Hindu (1996) and God as a Political Philosopher: Buddha's Challenge to Brahmanism (2001)* have been considered the first books are written by a Dalit scholar from the perspective of the political philosophy of Buddha.

Ambedkar's view on conversion once led him to question: does Hinduism give any mental and moral relief to the millions of the Backward Classes and Scheduled Castes (SCs)? Do Hindus expect these backward classes and the scheduled castes (SCs) to live under Hinduism, which gives them no promise of mental and moral relief? Such an expectation would be utter futility. Hinduism is floating on a volcano. Today it appears to be extinct, but it is not. It will become active once these mighty millions have become conscious of their degradation and that it is mainly due to the source of philosophy of the Hindu religion (ibid.).

4.4 Dalit Identity

Several scholars have discussed Dalits and their identity. Shah (2001) also discusses "Dalit identity and politics" and presents the idea of Mahatma Gandhi, an ardent champion for removing untouchability within the Hindu *Chatur-Varna* framework, who named the untouchable as the 'Harijan' man of God. The denomination got in usage 1931 amid conflicts between Gandhi and Ambedkar on the issue of political representation to Dalits based on a separate community, distinct from Hindus.

Gandhi explained the term Harijan in detail merely to give them an equal social identity within the Hindu caste framework or outside of it. He stated that the untouchables toil and moil and dirty their hands so that others may live in comfort and cleanliness. Others who in turn have delighted in suppressing them; he emphasised that Hindus are solely responsible for all the shortcomings and faults that we mostly put down those stigmas and sufferings at the door of those untouchables to be suffered for years (ibid. 25). The dignity should be given and bestowed upon the untouchable group to recognise their appropriate role in doing menial tasks and maintaining the social framework.

There have been several studies on caste in Indian society, and these include Risley, The People Of India (1915); Ghurye, Caste and Race in India (1932) and Caste and Class in India (1957); F. G. Bailey, Caste, And Economic Frontier (1957); Marriott, Caste Ranking And Community Structure In Five Regions Of India And Pakistan (1960); Hutton, Caste In India: Its Nature, Function And Origin (1961); Srinivas, Caste In Modern India And Other Essays (1962); Karve, Hindu Society; An Interpretation (1968); Mandelbaum, *Society In India, Vol.1: Continuity And Changes, Vol. II: Change And Continuity* (1970); Dumont's Homohierarchicus, The Caste System And Its Implications (1970); the work of Andre Betille, Y. Singh and Dipankar Gupta; and Ahamad, *Caste And Social Stratification Among Muslims* (1973).

Freeman (1997) has written an extensive and well-versed life history of untouchables. In this work, he sketches the life history of a person belonging to the Bauri caste-based in the state of Orissa. The untouchable's name is Muli, who lives three miles away from Bhubneshwar. In his work in *Untouchable,* James Freeman gives an exciting account of a person belonging to the Bauri caste. He states how they deal with a dead body and writes about their belief in a ghost or soul remaining in existence even after the death of family members.

He introduces this caste's association with the stigma attached to them, as "stigmatised from birth as spirituality defiling and therefore potential polluters of "clean" high caste people. India's untouchables lived for centuries in segregated hamlets and villages. High castes denied them the use of public wells and entry to schools, shops, and high-caste shrines. They forced them to perform the most despised and defiling jobs of their society: exhausting unskilled physical labour scavenging, cleaning latrines, and carrying off dead animals" (ibid.).

Many Westerners have written about India's problems of modernisation, urbanisation, poverty, population growth, and political stability, usually from western points of view or from those of high-level Indian administrators and politicians. Few studies on social change probe were deep enough to reveal what ordinary Indians think about their transition to modernity, especially in reference to untouchables. However, at least a handful of studies represent the complex and suppressed voices of Dalits. One can imagine Dalits and Dalits among Dalits, i.e., scavengers, as a particular category.

4.5 Health and Occupation

Park and Park (1991) identified the following determinants of health:

1. Environment
2. Life style
3. Socio-economic conditions
4. Health & family welfare services
5. Other factors

The most significant factor here is the socioeconomic condition of any particular community, and Dalits are situated at the lowest socioeconomic level. There is, therefore, an urgent need to examine the health issues of Dalit scavengers especially. The studies on Dalits and scavengers have some drawbacks; however, they failed in the application of the objectives laid down by the International Epidemiological Association (1973):

1. To describe the distribution and size of disease problems in human populations.
2. To identity etiological factors in the pathogenesis of the disease.
3. To provide the data essential to the planning, implementation and evaluation of services for the prevention, control and treatment of disease and the setting up of priorities among these services.

There is a vast gulf in health status among upper castes and Dalits in general and Dalits and scavengers in particular. People constantly exposed to filthy environments have a higher risk to his health than one who never gets exposed to such conditions. Understanding touchability and untouchability has to be concisely understood to improve the perception of the difference in the health status of different caste groups.

The distinction between touchability and untouchability is well explained by Anand (2000). Anything that may be touched by any portion of the body yet does not injure it mistakenly is considered touchable. Untouchable refers to anything that comes into contact with any part of the body and causes harm. These can easily be distinguished as "fire, electricity, too much exposure to sun rays, radioactive material, poisons, certain bacteria, some inorganic acids and alkalis, poisonous gases, bites by poisonous insects and animals and contact with some poisonous plants".

No particular human being falls in the category of untouchability. By touching a person, nobody gets sick or harmed or polluted.

Caste is an important factor that differentiates the health status of different caste groups but not necessarily the only factor if we see the work done by a Dalit is more demanding than the work of the upper castes. The harsh working conditions of Dalits are not found among the other upper caste groups. How is it that a person, who can break stones with a hammer all day in the scorching sun, could be incapable of holding a sword (one-fourth of the hammer) and fighting with the enemy? However, not allowing arms to Shudras or Dalits was a different intrigue of the Brahmins (Anand 2000).

It seems ridiculous to differentiate a person having the same blood, same biological organ, and similar race – yet he is treated indifferently and harshly. The living conditions of Dalits and Dalit scavengers are not the outcome of their action, but instead seem and appears a planned and ritually categorically framed ruse.

A scavenger has to create alternatives to cope with everyday life's working conditions. The use of alcohol in heavy doses becomes the necessary need of their working condition and thus for livelihood. Carrying nightsoil cleaning toilets/latrines every day threaten one's health; infections such as tuberculosis, malaria and skin diseases get transmitted through exposure to excreta.

The field of study for this work is a settlement of scavengers belonging to ex-untouchables, popularly known as Mehtar/Bhangi but locally known as *Hadi*. The use of alcohol and locally made liquors are very high among all sections and age groups, intending to seek respite from working conditions, poverty and related problems.

Public health issues have been one of the most neglected sectors. Ever since the liberalisation of the Indian economy, one has to illustrate the issue of Dalits in the context of the new economic policy moving towards the privatisation" of all public sectors. Even after five decades of independence, the reality of the constitution has not become a part of the ordinary Indian. One could reasonably expect to improve the condition of Dalits who still do not have space to say or voice before an upper (*dvija*) born caste member.

In this scenario, while increasing the location of health investment, in India, it has been one of the world's lowest public health investment countries. Worse still, during the nineties, as a percentage of GDP (Gross Domestic Product), public health funding declined from 1.3 per cent in 1990 to 0.9 per cent in 1999. An in

Differences in Health Status among Socio-Economic Groups

Serial No.	**Indicator**	**Infant mortality/ 1000**	**Under-5 mortality/ 1000**	**% children underweight**
1	**India**	70	94.9	47
2	**Scheduled Castes**	83	119.3	53.5
3	**Scheduled Tribes**	84.2	126.6	55.9
4	**Other Disadvantaged**	76	103.1	47.3
5	**Others**	61.8	82.6	41.1

Source: National Health Policy 2001, Delhi Science Forum, New Delhi

The poor level of health indicator among Dalits (SCs) is exceptionally high compared to the general population, and infant mortality among SCs is second highest after Scheduled Tribes (STs). Nonetheless, we could get infant mortality statistics for Dalits engaged in scavenging and dirty jobs (based on different caste categories). In that situation, the statistics may show a drastically different picture.

CHAPTER THREE

THE SOCIO-DEMOGRAPHIC AND ECONOMIC PROFILE OF HADIS

1. An overview of the city of Bokaro

On April 1, 1991, the district of Bokaro was formed by separating one sub-division, Chas, from the Dhanbad district and another, Bermo, from the Giridih district. Dhanbad is on the district's western border, Hazaribagh is on the district's eastern border, Purulia is on the district's southern border, and Giridih is on the district's northern border.

India's largest steel complex is located along the Dhanbad Ranchi highway, close to the west of India's major iron and steel mills. The factory will be the country's first Swadeshi plant (usually manufactured in India). Steel plant to be created with the highest level of indigenization in terms of equipment, materials, and know-how! As a result, this project represents a significant shift from the previous reliance on foreign sources for know-how and consulting, design and equipment, supervision, and erection to virtually complete self-sufficiency and trust.

The city's broad rolling geography littered by graded valleys and flowing streams, is typical of the Chotanagpur Plateau. In this context, a new metropolis with a strong multi-dimensional economic base has grown into a regional urban centre with a population of roughly 0.1 million people drawn from all over the country, giving the city the character of a mini-Bharat, India. The Bokaro Steel Plant (BSL) started producing ingot steel in October 1972 and produced 1.7 million tonnes in 1978.

BSL now produces almost 4.5 million tonnes of crude steel and 3.8 million tonnes of hot and cold rolled products, making it a crown gem of Steel Authority of India Limited (SAIL). Bokaro has established itself as a respected maker of continuous cast slabs. Railways, Defence, the white goods sector, tube producers, barrel and bitumen, Liquefied Petroleum Gas (LPG), the cycle industry, the cane industry, and many other customers are served by Bokaro Steel. Bokaro Steel City was envisaged in 1959 as the fourth integrated steel facility in the public sector. The Union of Soviet Socialist Republics (USSR) assisted in constructing the Bokaro Steel Plant, which began in 1965.

Nearby localities are home to central coalfields. For the staff of the factories, Bokaro City was developed to provide housing and other community facilities. Bokaro City is located on the southern side of the Garga River, one of its tributaries to the Damodar River, which meanders along the city's southern and eastern fringes. The city is bounded north by the Parasnath Hills and the south by the Satanpur hillocks located just beyond the Garga River.

1.1 The Town

The township, which has a stunning natural setting and mountainous resources, has the best resources in the city. The city's planning reflects a long-term ecological system and marketplace arrangements appropriate for modern life. The educational system is essential in introducing the best-behaved students to the country, and this group of graduates has excelled in the most significant Indian institutions.

1.1.1 Bokaro *Ispat Pustakalaya*

The town's library has a collection of over 40,000 books that meets the reading requirements of the people in the township. The planning included creating and teaching a habit of reading among residents, though it is limited to the employed people to the steel plant and reside nearby.

1.1.2 City Park

Bokaro has a well-maintained City Park with an artificial lake. Recently three artificial islands have also been created. A Biological Park named after Jawaharlal Nehru with various animals and birds and a modern aquarium is another attraction. The park is at a distance of four kilometres close to the Hadi Cooli settlement that allows Hadi families to visit on some occasions for an outing with family and friends.

The Bokaro district website refers to two sources of historical accounts, The Settlement Report for Manbhum (1928) and the District Gazetteer for Dhanbad (1964) are invaluable resources available to trace the history of the areas falling within the Bokaro District Manual (1999). The early history of the greater part of the area is difficult to trace, as the present district formed out of a small and insignificant part of Manbhum. In the Settlement Report for Manbhum (1928), it has been stated that no rock inscriptions, copper plates or old coins got discovered during the survey and settlement operations. The oldest authentic documents produced were on paper and barely a hundred years old.

The district of Bokaro was earlier a part of the district of Manbhum. Manbhum derived its name from Raja Man Singh, who received this territory as a gift from the emperor Akbar. Later, the extremely vast and far-flung district of Manbhum was divided into Birbhum, Manbhum and Singhbhum. Later still, on October 25th 1956, Dhanbad was created on the recommendation of the State Reconstruction Commission. The district of Dhanbad consisted of two subdivisions, namely Dhanbad and Baghmara. On April 1st, 1991, the Baghmara subdivision also known Chas became part of the Bokaro district. The area now forming part of Bokaro district was inhabited primarily by people of the Kolas race (Bokaro District Manual, 1999).

The Jains were the first civilisation in the area around 600 B.C. As revealed by Huein Tsang's (2006) Travel Accounts, which cites a large realm ruled by Sasanka, a Buddhist prosecutor, the Brahmins eclipsed the Jain domination around the seventh century A.D. After that, the Bhumij and the Mundari tribe eliminated the Brahmin culture.

Raja Man Singh led his army through Jharkhand from Bhagalpur to Midnapur, which is now part of West Bengal, during Akbar's reign. He may have travelled through the Bokaro district, according to reports (ibid). In fact, the area earned prominence and a spot on the Indian map when the Indian government decided in the early 1960s to build a modern public-sector steel plant with Soviet Russia's assistance. Indira Gandhi, India's Prime Minister, lay the foundation stone for what is now known as the Bokaro Steel Plant (BSL) in 1966.

In the early 1990s, a new horizon was opened when the Oil Natural Gas Corporation (ONGC) discovered a vast methane gas deposit in the Chandankyari area, which is part of the Bokaro district. According to reports, the ONGC has begun constructing a massive plant in the region that will progressively grow in size and importance beyond the current Bokaro Steel Plant.

1.1.3 The Natural Division

The district may be categorised into three natural formations:

i. Central Plateau.
ii. Lower Plateau.
iii. Domodar, Garga and Tenughat Valley.

1.1.4 The Climate and Rainfall

The climate of this region is sub-tropical and annual rainfall lies between a minimum of 157 cm to a maximum of 195 cm. The general temperature falls to a minimum of 2^0C during the winter and rises to a maximum of 45^0C in summer. The wind direction is from south-west to north-west. The district, falling in the tropical monsoon region, has three broadly pronounced seasons: i) Cool season: October to February; (ii) Hot season: March to May; and iii) Raining season: June to September.

The Damodar is the most important river of the Chotanagpur plateau. It rises in the Palamu district of Jharkhand and flows eastward between the plateau of Ranchi and Hazaribagh in Bokaro district. A dam has been constructed at Tenughat on the river Damodar that provides water to the Bokaro Steel Plant for its operation and for irrigation facilities.

Another river, the "Garga," also flows between Chas Municipality and BSC area. There is a small dam on the Garga river. Other small rivers of the district are the Gobai, which flows through Chandankiyari Block area, and Konar River in Gomia Block. The Bokaro district is mostly hilly and soil is generally shallow and infertile.

Hardly eight percent of total agricultural land is irrigated in the district; the majority of agriculture depends solely on the monsoon precipitation. In most areas, only marginal and sub-marginal farming is possible. The land use pattern of the district can thus be described as mostly monocropped and rainfed. Hills and forests cover it, and the soil is generally rocky and sandy. Only 39.21 percent of the total area of the district is presently under agriculture, the horticultural area is about 9.09 percent of the cultivable land. The main agricultural crops are rice and maize, while bajra, wheat, pulses and vegetables are also cultivated. A marginal portion of non-forest land,

Gair Majoorwa[1] (GM) lands, and Raiyati land is under horticulture and social forestry.

1.1.5 Irrigation

Since the topography of the district is hilly, there is not much scope for retaining the surface water. The other means of irrigation left in this area is in the exploitation of ground water, taking recourse to lift irrigation. Tank irrigation is quite popular in the district. After independence of India, it is during 1948 the Damodar Valley Corporation (DVC) and district authorities set up several water schemes. River irrigation schemes, open boring, tube wells and hand pumps have been installed in the recent past for amelioration of local population and their irrigation needs. The same system continues even after few decades afterwards the water supply is still dependent on DVC.

1.1.6 Mines and Minerals

The Bermo-Phurro – an area of Bokaro district known for its coalmines – coalfield area is entirely situated in this district and is rich in coal. Apart from coal, other minerals such as fire clay and limestone are commonly found. A number of quarries for the extraction of stone, stone boulders and production of stone chips are also being run.

1.1.7 Industries

The Bokaro district headquarters have occupied a very important role in the industrialisation of the Jharkhand state and the country as a whole since the establishment of the first steel plant in 1965. The fourth integrated steel plant in the public sector, Bokaro Steel Plant, started production in the 1970s with the collaboration of the Soviet Union. At present, production of steel is listed at 4 million tonnes, which will likely increase up to 10 million tonnes annually. Bokaro is thus stated to be India's largest industrial

---

[1] Gair Majoorwa is a kind of land in India that does not have a proper record in government land records. "Generally, some land is found that is neither owned by individuals nor by the government, known as "*Gair Majurwa Zameen*" (Lahiri-Dutt, Krishnan and Ahmed, 2012). Such lands can be used by government for community purposes and at times people also use them until government take over. The absence of *gair majurwa zameen* near Hadi Cooli also minimized their residential expansion and they got confined in the same land which was enough when the first settlers constructed their houses and settled down in the present Hadi Cooli" (Ziyauddin, 2017, unpublished).

complex; coal manufacture for the steel plant is supplied by different companies that washes and cleans the raw coals to be used in the steel plant (known as Washeries), and they are located at places like Dugdha, Kathara, Kargali etc. In addition, the Damodar Valley Corporation (DVC), a multipurpose project, produces power for the industrialisation of the district and the whole state of Jharkhand and West Bengal. Bokaro is a highly industrialised district due to the location of the steel plant at district headquarters, Bokaro. A series of small-scale industries have emerged in the industrial area of Bokaro, which cater to the needs of the Bokaro steel plant. Recently a Thermal Power Plant has emerged in Tenughat with a power generation of 440 MW. There are also two manufacturing industries located in the "Balidih" and "Jainamore" industrial areas respectively, both are auxiliaries to Bokaro Steel Plant.

1.2 Demographic Description

The total population of the Bokaro district is 145,723 which is divided into urban (593,129), and rural population (864,106) as according to the 1991 census. Out of the total population, the male population is 776,974 and female population is 680,261 of which Scheduled Castes (SCs) make up 158,616 and Schedule Tribes (STs) 160,617. But during the last two census enumeration, the population has increased drastically and in the 2001 census data, it had increased to 1,777,662 and in the next census survey, in 2011 census of India, it reached 2,062,330. The decadal growth of the population of Bokaro was found to be 22.11 percent during 1991-2001 but it declined to 16.01 percent in 2011. The density of the district per square kilometre was 508 in 1991 (Census of India), which has increased to 621 in 2001 and 715 in 2011 (Census of India). In the district, the number of women per thousand men has increased from 865 in 1991 to 894 in 2001, and quite recently to 922. The total number of people in the work force involved in agriculture is 31,266. In the last census enumeration report of 2011, the SCs population in the district rose to 299,227 out of the total population of 144,930.

The Bokaro district consists of two sub-divisions, eight Development Blocks and 136 Panchayats with 639 villages in number. The district is densely populated with a population density of 662 per square kilometre.

Now the focus shall turn to the Chas township area and its total population distribution. As of the District Primary Abstract Census of 1991, the total population of the Chas Municipal Corporation Area is 65,207, in comparison to the Chas Block population of 565,290. The number of Dalits

(SCs) in the Chas Municipal area is 6,624 of which 3,489 are male and 3,135 are female. There is an increasing tendency seen in the overall population of the township to migrate. On the other hand, the total population of Chas Block is 565,290 of which Scheduled Castes number 66,782.

The Sadar sub-division of the Chas municipality, is situated in the district headquarters, Bokaro There are two blocks under this sub-division. One is Mufassil Block in Chas itself and another is Chandankyari Block which is 30 kilometres away from the sub-divisional headquarters with 43 Panchayats. The total population of this sub division is 741,921.

2. Description of the Research Field

2.1 Chas

The purpose behind the selection of the research field Chas, a Municipal Corporation area and a part of the Bokaro Steel City urban agglomeration in terms of the urban population census, has various bases and understandings.

As of now, the population distribution of Dalits in the Chas municipal area has been given. The most significant factor is the surrounding area of Chas. Chas has a good number of Marwari communities, followed by Sikhs and Hindu "Baniyas" who hold the key to the whole/entire sector of business transactions within the region. Chas is not a newly developed township but it was around before the establishment of the Bokaro Steel Plant. The area surrounding the main market of Chas is for a large majority inhabited by the business community. A region having previously been a part of the Purulia district of West Bengal, some local inhabitants speak Bengali, which has also influenced the local dialect. One can notice the use of Bengali words typically in the local dialects among the non-Bengali speaking population as a definite marker of the area's past relationship with West Bengal.

Due to lack of the sewerage system, the community, i.e. the *Hadi*s, who are traditionally engaged in the manual cleaning of waste materials and latrines, have better prospects of carrying out their occupation. The area covering the Chas municipality is being taken care of by the Mines Area Development Authority, popularly known as MADA, which has its office in the Dhanbad district.

The other factor which led the researcher to select this area was the population of "Hadi Cooli" who are primarily engaged in scavenging and cleaning latrines. Despite being the nearest settlement to the main market, the housing conditions, sanitation facilities and environmental surroundings are much worse than other, further away, settled communities. They don't have a single public tap or hand pump or place where they can bathe or wash clothes unlike other castes in neighbouring settlements. The tyranny does not end there since they wash clothes and take baths in the same ponds used afterwards as toilets. All these facts were observed during the pilot visit to the area. These observations, based on non-participation of the researcher, encouraged the undertaking of research on this particular community. Chas has attracted a good number of migrants that have densified the population of Bokaro district.

2.2 Household Population of the Hadi Caste

According to the estimation of local leaders and older responsible members of the Hadi community, there are 48 families of the Hadi caste who reside in the Hadi Cooli ("Cooli" is a term for mohalla). This mohalla is just a few metres away from the main market of Chas town. The process of constructing new houses has expanded the settlement to those areas of Chas, which had been agricultural ten years previously. The Hadi Cooli is geographically surrounded by other mohallas on three fronts or sides and in the eastern part runs a *Joria* (*Nala* or stream) which carries and collects waste (i.e. from residents' houses and small industries), through a drain of the Chas township. South of the Hadi Cooli is the main market, known as *Mahabir Chowk* main market. In the northwestern part are the settlements of the Muslim community, and the northeast is populated by the Bauri caste, known as Bauri Cooli. The Bauri caste pertains to "scheduled" communities now mainly engaged in collecting and selling waste materials (Kabadi).

This area is characterised by well-separated settlements in terms of the communities settled there. These mohallas start from the Muslim mohalla and are followed by others, namely; Ansari Mohalla, Ansar Nagar, Sultan Nagar, Azad Nagar, Ghaush Nagar, and Bharra Basti. These mohallas are inhabited by the Muslims, the majority of them consisting of outsiders or migrants throughout the Jharkhand and Bihar. Only three small Coolis (Mohallas) are in highly Muslim populated settlements.

The most striking feature is that all these Coolis are Dalit-populated and most are engaged in menial and lowly occupations in the social hierarchy. Hadi, Bauri, and Shakara Cooli are the three mohallas, respectively. The other caste communities living in the same localities for generations now significantly require rigorous research which is not touched on deeply in the present text.

2.2.1 Bauri Cooli

The Bauri Cooli is estimated to have around 200 families. The majority of the population is engaged in Kabadi works, or as rickshaw pullers, and vendors in different parts of Chas township. A few work as casual labourers. The housing condition is not good, even this community has Kutcha houses. Only five to ten percent have pucca and semi pucca buildings. Traditionally this community is not involved in "polluted" occupations. They have been doing paid labour-based jobs, either in the agricultural fields or in houses or at construction sites. The Bauri level of literacy is very low. During group discussions, it was observed that school education is out of their reach.

A few families however are well educated because of their landholdings in past generations. The Bauri caste is listed in the census of India among the Scheduled Castes. They primarily speak Bengali. The children of their families are engaged in rag picking. This was discovered during the study: that in the whole township area, the children of the Bauri caste collect garbage and pick-up usable items from the streets and different corners of the town.

2.2.2 Shakara Cooli

This is also a mohalla of "scheduled" communities who are mainly engaged in different daily-based earning jobs. The Shakara Cooli is engaged in their traditional occupation of "Pot-making" (i.e. thathera). Before the construction of the steel plant, they were successful in marketing their product because there was enough demand in the market; this occupation had good sales and profits. Chas was only a small township through which one National Highway crosses to Dhanbad on the one side and Purulia, a district of West Bengal, on the other, while the third road goes to Ranchi, the state capital of Jharkhand. These three main highways meet at Chas, which is three kilometres away from Hadi Cooli. So it has got a good network of roadway facilities. After the establishment of Bokaro Steel Plant, most of the goods were transported to and from the steel plant through these roads. In the process, Chas developed a big sector of employment in heavy motor part shops, mechanical oriented workshops and garages. This opened up new employment opportunities for thousands of people. Interestingly, Muslims dominate the sector of repairing and mechanical works as has also been pointed in the Sachar Committee Report (2006).

The reason behind this dynamic developmental change in Chas gives us a base to understand the decline in the market demand of locally made metallic pots by the Shakara caste. Through the process of urbanisation, many new well-maintained markets and shopping complexes have developed. Undoubtedly, this process pushed this community to stop their traditionally based business, because they could not offer the new standards of market trends. In this context, the demerits of urbanisation have been proved worthy to demolish the well-maintained and highly demanded products of the local market, produced by this community.

So the well-settled community changed occupation from the making and selling of aluminium, copper, and brass pots to collecting the Kabadi of these metals.

Children of the Shakara community could also be seen in the streets, collecting all waste stuffs from dustbins. These rag pickers, who are in the age group of four-five years, start working as rag pickers to support their family by improving the total family income.

The nature of the families is nuclear. This fact was explored through the informal discussion with the families from the same caste. Senior community fellows also consulted on this issue had similar views.

The general views expressed in the in-depth group discussion held at this Cooli suggest that most of the Kabadi works in Chas town area reach this mohalla. This is because the entire mohalla is engaged in the same job, the reason is non-availability of other option. They harbour deep anger towards state policy and sometimes feel that they themselves are also responsible for the deterioration of their living conditions. Few families, to whom the researcher could manage to talk, found that there are few households who do not own their house. The other side of this story is that some families sold their own houses due to acute poverty. Now they are staying in the same house as tenants.

The Shakara Cooli has a homogenous population in terms of caste and occupation. Men and women are found to be engaged in the same occupation. This is not by choice but due to the social, political and economic changes that have enforced this community to stay in this hazardous and stigmatised occupation. Girls are more vulnerable and are being sexually abused. Early marriages of girls lead to increased vulnerability.

2.3 Housing and Living Conditions

Except for two or three, all houses in the Hadi Cooli are kutcha houses. Whatever the structures of their house may be, they own their houses, which is the most interesting question or issue. One typical observation that could be illustrated is regarding the houses they have. Generally, they don't have more than two rooms. People would be happier in the community if they possessed a house with two rooms and a veranda. Most of the houses are very small in size. Rooms are very congested and there is no ventilation except in Pucca houses, and the floor is made of soil. The distinct observation regarding the door is the height of their doors. The vertical length/height of the doors is so low that one has to bend one's head to enter the house. The famous saying, that lower castes or untouchables were supposed to keep their doors short in heights that they would be obliged to show deference to the upper castes (in bowing their heads) when they come outside/out of their houses/of the front door, almost seems true.

The number of people per room is around five or more, and the rooms are small in size and congested. The concept of separate cooking space does not exist; the (living) conditions are such that they cannot even think about it because many of them have only a single room. The reason for having small rooms is that they do not have any more land around the place. A few decades ago, the Hadi Cooli were really at the outskirts of Chas, but as soon as the process of urbanisation picked up momentum, the population started settling down leaving the Hadi Cooli in the middle of the whole area. All Hadi families are dependent on a public tap, situated at a distance of around half a kilometre from their settlement.

In fact, the Bauri Cooli do not have a proper source of drinking water either. This is only found in the Shakara Cooli, where some families have a hand pump and well, only because these families had owned large areas of agricultural land around ten-fifteen years previously. These sources are as old as their past history. So, all of them carry water from the public tap which is at the middle of the market of Chas near the bus stop.

The public tap is just beside the drain flowing through the Chas market. No doubt, the water generally flows into the tap for the whole day, but the spot where it lies is just beside the drain (Joria).

One can see the long queue every time they go over there to collect water. Women and girls have to carry water on their heads every day, in the morning and evening. This is a major job for them and it takes around five hours. The rest of the day's hours are for cooking and collecting or managing cooking fuel.

Though Bokaro is one of the richest coal reserves and mining districts *of* India, the people who live in the region have no access to coal for fuel. There is no any coal depot for people to access which provides cheap fuel. The crisis has created a high demand for coal in the illegal market. The unemployed population of the surrounding areas, where coal is mined, collect coal illegally and sell it from door to door in the township but also more in rural areas. This has given way to illegal mining by different "Coal Mafias" and local criminals who sell it illegally on a large scale. Thousands of people around the town have made it a major source of livelihood, by selling the coal in different colonies of the district. But these are not members of the Hadi Cooli. When the need arises to check illegal mining from the district administration, the majority of the lower-class population face an acute crisis because they don't have any other source of fuel. Hadis especially are not economically well off enough to afford fuel at a high cost. However, they are forced to purchase it anyway because there is simply no alternative. Kerosene oil is provided by the Public Distribution System (PDS) at a lower price but most of them do not get it. Many of the families do not have a Red Card (given to BPL families). A few of them have ration cards but they do not have access to the different goods provided by the state, the reason being non-availability of the goods in the PDS centre.

Nobody can blame the people who are engaged in coal selling, without ignoring the fact that without the involvement of police or administration the illegal sale and mining of coal and mining wouldn't be possible.

The logic behind this explanation lies in understanding the proportion of household expenditure on fuel in comparison to the other expenses: fuel heavily diminishes/reduces the total income of the households.

There are a few families who have toilets in their houses. They even do not have any public or common toilet around the mohalla /Cooli. The sense of common space is there because all of them use the common area for toilet purposes, which is the nearest field to the Joria. The Joria is a stream, which comes out of Chas collecting all the waste of the town that flows just behind (on the eastern side) the Hadi Cooli. A person other than from this community cannot spend more than a few minutes near the Joria because it smells too bad. But some of the families wash clothes and bathe in that slow stream. The bathing and washing of clothes are also done in the pond which is at a distance of a half kilometre from the Hadi Cooli. In fact, most of the members of "scheduled" communities have access to this pond. This is because the other ponds no longer has water due to the lowering down of ground water all over the district.

None of the families has in-house toilet facilities except one. This is a far and distant dream when one does not even have drinking water in the mohalla/Cooli.

Every caste group tries to improve its social status in society through the help of economic improvement. The notion of "pollution and purity" is only found when a caste group has substantial surplus to sustain their livelihood. This concept is used only to monopolise the economy as a whole where the share of the surplus amount is distributed among certain privileged/elite groups only: There is always a creation of new groups who can do the service in minimum wages. Religion is used to strengthen the argument given in this process of exploitation. The crux of Marxian philosophy on religion seems suitable where it is said: "Religion [...] is the opium of the people" (Marx and Davis, 1994).

In the present context, Dalits, especially the *Dalit* scavengers, are the most deprived section of the population. Hence, the purpose behind the argument of this study is to show that economy has the power to maintain the hegemony of concepts such as pollution and purity.

There have been several attempts to provide toilet facilities and sanitation but they have always lacked a need-based approach. The whole settlement does its best to use the Joria and the natural ponds.

2.4 Electricity

Most of the families do have electricity. However, ways of accessing it differ. Those who are 'better' than other members of the community have legally accessed electricity, but a few of them divert it illegally. Some pay fifty rupees per month to the electricity department.

The duration of the power supply is generally eighteen hours per day although there is no guarantee. The use of electricity is only for lighting purposes, since they do not own modern luxury items. Popular recreation in their life is simply talking and chatting with each other and watching films at the nearest theatre, the Chandra Cinema.

2.5 Occupational Observation

All the families of the Hadi Cooli are from similar caste and socio-economic groups. They belong to "scheduled" communities engaged in polluted occupations. Dalits are a 'polluted group' in the Hindu caste hierarchy but only very few caste groups are engaged in so-called "degraded" or "polluted" jobs.

The notion of "purity/pollution" is very harsh and crude; especially for those castes engaged in the "polluted" occupations. A fair portion of religious communities in India discriminate in this way. If one thinks of changing the meaning or importance placed on birth identity, *even then* such families or individuals will not be able to change their status. At times, the feeling is that there is no need to change caste identity or to ever try and defy caste boundaries. This attitude develops after a long perpetual and perennial cycle of degraded life. The "polluted" have limited livelihood options. The sense of job security among the youth is very high They are interested in other types of work but these are not available. This idea was grasped during the Focus Group Discussion (FGDs) with the youth of the same community.

The major problem noticed was the involvement in gambling of the whole community including members of the Bauri and Shakara groups. The reason for this is the non-availability of job opportunities also the sense of work security in that they can carry out their traditional occupation in the respective areas. Those in the whole settlement of these Dalits (including the Bauri and Shakara Cooli) are very fond of card playing and gambling. Even if they don't have money, this is a favourite game for passing the time. The kind of social pressure which could minimise this 'social evil' is absent because all the age groups are involved in the same activity. No legal action is taken because the local police personnel are content to charge a weekly or monthly sum and then leave them to it. This has encouraged the local mafia to sell locally made liquor illegally in the Cooli. Whenever the police create problems, the mafia pays a fixed to the police. Few members of the Bauri caste expressed their anxieties about their helpless condition. Many of the responsible and concerned community members were of the view that the selling of illegal liquor in the Cooli should stop; even adolescents have become daily consumers. In this situation, their condition worsens because even if they earn some money every day, it is spent on these activities.

The level of social interaction with other communities is limited. There are no upper caste families in the surrounding area. The Muslim community does not follow or practise the theory of pollution and purity but the essence of this notion exists somewhere in their practical life. However, the surrounding population helps Hadis stay and breathe freely. If there had been a member of an upper Hindu caste next door, for example, the social environment would have been different.

This is an important aspect with which we can see the social stigma attached to this caste and their special occupation to assess their living and social condition.

Due to the increase in urban population around this settlement, density has also increased although the level of social interaction is decreasing. This phenomenon leads to a positive change when we compare the inevitable rigid attachment of pollution and purity with the special castes. Fewer interactions, less identification, lead to a decline in social pressure. The change in urban society from collective consciousness to individual consciousness in a way weakens the hierarchical set up of the Hindu caste system.

One mere observation is in the dress pattern of this community. If they dress well during leisure time, it may be difficult to identify them as fellow members of the Hadi caste. They are very conscious of dress style.

One question remains about their traditional occupation. Why are they not able to change occupation? If they want to, then what are the factors which force them to continue this work?

The first explanation depends on the understanding of the 'special' occupation. The family and social institution to carry out their traditional occupation are socialising them. The level of awareness is more or less good. Few people expressed the view that education could be used as an instrument to improve the social status within the social structure, but the existing social structure neither allows nor encourages this. The level of income is very low or meagre which makes them think of it as supplementary support system for new income. Lack of educational facilities is also responsible for their deteriorating condition. The permanent 'strike' by upper caste groups through various media has been a catalyst for continuity of the same occupation.

It is important to address the factor of the sewerage system. This is basically a very complex question about whether a township has a proper sewerage system or not. But most of the drains are handled by this caste in the Chas area. They are the local inhabitants of this region and place. I can illustrate the fact that even before the existence of the Bokaro Steel Plant, they were in the same position. In the agriculture-based society, they also performed "degraded" work. Not one of them had any land in the past nor do they possess any in the present era.

A twenty-five-year-old told me that the situation has changed now. At least now they can drink water or eat food in the different hotels and dhabas in the market. One generation ago, they suffered from tremendous stigma throughout their life. They were not allowed to do anything in public places. In the main market of Chas, adjacent to their Cooli, there are hundreds of families (Bengali upper caste), who never allowed these Dalits to enter their houses. But now the situation has changed. Some women from the Dalit community now undertake domestic work as cleaners in these houses.

This is a kind of change in the social set-up where at least they can interact with others and earn some amount of money, even if at very low wages.

The status of women can be seen only according to their earnings and at times this becomes the overriding factor which situates the status of women as house-bound in the home. The field observation aims to understand and look into the deeper meaning of being a woman in the Hadi and Dalit communities, and their importance within the family and kingroup in particular. The men always make the decisions but women's views are also taken into account on every occasion.

One can also illustrate the economic structure and mode of earning of the community. The economic structure is based largely on a single occupation. There is no demand for monetary investment but the acquisition of skill is necessary. Women are usually always engaged in domestic work, so the concentration of men in these occupations is very high. The availability of alternative jobs for women is limited; they can also be found engaged in different occupations but the earnings are not satisfactory.

In spite of schools of thought advocating for the liberation of women, they are always dependent on men because they have not been provided opportunities to work.

2.6 An Outline of the Study Area

Currently, this region/area is in the process of change and transformation. Transformation in itself carries complex ideas but here what is perceived is that this process is having the phenomena of social and economic change. Transformation means the total or partial change in something already existing. The life of the Dalits in a way has some influence on the major Muslim community in the area. The Muslim area consists of a dense population of local inhabitants, though being a part of the Bokaro Steel City, it has attracted large numbers of migrants from Bihar and other states around the country.

It was found that the area was congested and had narrow streets and roads passing through the different Cooli. The new construction of the main road crossing over from the Mohalla has given a new shape to the whole area comprising entire mohallas.

Around eight Registered Medical Practitioners (RMPs) could be seen in the whole locality; these RMPs are always freely accessible at any time of day.

Private doctors' practices and clinics/nursing homes are being set up in all parts of Chas and Bokaro in general; in particular, there are a few places" where only these "private" institutions are located.

Children are always exposed to dirt and waste materials. The drains are not covered in the Bauri Cooli but the Hadi Cooli does not have even any proper drainage. Many households who dig their drains in the earth and dispose waste-water into that. In the process, they clean out and throw the wastewater in the open drains passing through the main road crossing through this the area. It is not surprising to see women washing cooking utensils at the doorstep of houses where all the waste water is logged.

The process of disinvestment of the public sector unit in the hand of private ownership has tremendous influence on the small business sector of Bokaro. Particularly, since the National Democratic Alliances (NDA) government has come in to power, this process has been rapid. Motor vehicle and motor mechanics-related businesses have also been impacted, because roadways are now used to transport most of the goods to and from the steel plant. After general observation of and discussion with the local businesses it was found that ever since SAIL set up the Voluntary Retirement Scheme (VRS), forced scrutiny has created a sense of insecurity which has compelled the people to slow down purchasing. Many employees of the steel plant will return to their hometown or area of origin after retirement. Hindustan Steel limited (HSL) is just about to close its unit. HSL is run from the Bokaro Steel Plant (BSL) premises which has done too much scrutiny according to the directed policy of central government.

BSL is the most profitable of the SAIL units, yet it has been declared a sick unit.

2.7 Perceptions of Hadis about themselves

In general, there is a trend among the population of feeling segregated from others. They do not interact with others because of the fact that they are members of the "polluted" caste. Still, they know that they have an important function to perform in society.

The stigma attached to their special occupation also influences their other activities. They attend all the special occasions and festivals celebrated by the caste. The new generation, those below the age of thirty, has a different perception about their lifestyle. They do not want to be obliged to any other caste groups and communities. They also want to enjoy their life in a free environment, and be able to breathe openly.

One may not be able to identify them if they dress unlike what is stereotypical of their caste. The other communities also have the same view about their dressing style. Most of them do the same job but in the evening, especially the youth, dress well and sit around the main market, and can also be found gathering in the nearest market "Mahabir Chowk". But then, the daily work routine resumes in the early morning and they search of a refreshment. Breakfast is generally not available in the early morning, so they start their day without food and go to their own area to see if there is any chance of getting work.

Every Friday is a special occasion: the day a new movie is released in the nearest cinema. The cinema hall is at a distance of less than a kilometre. The researcher tried to observe the crowd in this same cinema hall, known as the "Chandra Cinema"; most of the youth attend for the evening show. It is the major source of entertainment among the youth of the Hadi caste.

The dowry system is practised and it is found not only in Hadi but also Bauri and Shakara families. The majority of people are of the view that it is a social evil and an oppressive system, but they continue to follow the system because of the social pressure created by the brides' families.

Politically, Hadis are not attached to any political party; they follow whoever comes to the community and makes a series of commitments and promises. During the Focus Group Discussion, the major need and demand that was desired by the community members was that of school infrastructure. Every parent should be able to fulfil their desire of sending their children to school. The process of recruiting teachers for the school would be undertaken with community consultation: the teachers should be recruited from the community itself, so that the levels of classroom discrimination are minimised.

This method or approach will also give the children a feeling of being equal to others, which will serve to enhance the process of socialisation of the children and provide space for personal development. The level of motivation among community members to send their children to school is not low but rather is hindered by the non-availability of schools in the locality. There is a school just near the Hadi Cooli, but teachers there discriminate between students. They give less attention to the children who need the most care and attention. The middle school is in the middle of the Muslim mohalla and no more than a few students attend regularly. In other words, the majority of the students attending this school come from the Muslim families of the locality, not from the *Hadi* Cooli caste.

With discrimination is an issue, the feeling of inferiority among the Hadi students is high. They feel themselves to be separated, segregated and marginalised. In the process, schools do not represent a safe social space for them to interact with others, which can influence parents in deciding whether to send their children to school. The state goes by the criterion of distance and population. In this criterion, there is one state-run primary school, middle school and high school, but these are not accessible to them, when really special attention should be given to their educational attainment in particular.

The primary school is very near to the Hadi Cooli; why is it then that this community's children are not registered? The school is located on the bank of the *Joria* (*Nala or stream*), which flows on the eastern side of the Hadi Cooli. There are two rooms and a veranda, which is of *pucca* construction – this refers to buildings which are of flimsy construction. There are vacancies for two teachers, but only one teacher is posted, so the teacher is not able to provide proper guidance and education to all. The majority of the students are from the Bauri and Shakara castes and also from the Muslim community. The tendency of being used to getting exploited also worsens the condition of Dalits at school. The Hadis are always asked to stay away from others. Even a few Bauri caste members were heard saying that they cannot interact with Hadis, because they are engaged in "unclean occupation".

The school has no drinking water facility. In fact, one public hand pump was set up a few years ago, but it is no longer functional. The significant impression was that no publicly made construction or establishment for the welfare of the poor is well maintained. The main challenge is the rethinking of the future maintenance of such establishments. Even if there is a need to spend ten rupees on repair work, no one bothers. Community involvement is very important in the process of maintenance. In the present context of the debate, the hand pumps are not always maintained and fall into disrepair over time. The already constructed school building is no longer maintained. This is the scenario of a town where a proper chair is not available in any of the schools. Students bring their own stuff – small clothes and plastic sheets – to sit on in the classroom. The number of students from the Hadi Cooli is never more than ten; even those who attend do not come regularly because of the negative response and treatment they receive.

The name "Hadi Cooli" is derogatory in itself: if a person says that he/she is from the Hadi Cooli, other would usually choose to avoid them.

The consensus among the Hadi caste members was that they should have a separate school that every child could attend regularly. The perception of a child develops only from this age. The very process of socialisation starts after the birth of a child but the significant learning stage starts when children interact with their peers. They develop the perception of belonging to a particular family, which has a caste identity. That caste identity provides a platform to the growing individual and every child is trained in the family in such a manner, where they have to carry the status quo of their caste.

The middle school is located in an area dominated by the Muslim community. The reality is that the majority of its students are from the same community because it is Urdu medium school. Hence, most of the Dalit students go to other schools, which are run by different organisations and individuals. One of them is *Shishu Vidya Mandir*, an associated branch of Rashtriya Swanyam Sangh (RSS). Even there, hardly any children from the Hadi or Bauri castes are registered.

Talking about high school seems useless. Very few students manage to go to high school. The problem is not only with the family or familial background but also with a lack of motivation and awareness. There is hardly any families where the parents are keen to force their children into higher education. There are too many complexities surrounding their livelihood and life. The most recurring question was, what they will do if they go into higher education? There is no surety of any government job. How will an educated person feel when he/she doesn't get any opportunities? Further, education will not lead to any change in social status; they will still be known as members of a "polluted" community.

The other demotivating factor concerning school attendance is the school environment. Teachers are also role models for caste-based discrimination, because they promote the same ideas about caste structure that they have themselves learnt/internalised in their own upbringing. The larger population does not suffer from caste-based exploitation but Dalits of this occupational category do. Frustration with and towards state policy is very high and the main problem lies in the issue of awareness. Few of them are vocal or have tried to access schemes at the block development office level (a block is a unit of governance in each district through all schemes and programmes are to be implemented in a district). They do not know about the schemes for Dalits that try to promote the social status and aim at alleviating the poverty of these lower caste communities. Mediators or agents appear to be quite an important link between common and less educated people and the government officials. So many things come in the way of accessing anything. Schooling is not the priority of Hadi caste members because the search for employment starts anew every morning and ends with some rupees in the hand in the evening or night. However, a few households have provided their inclination towards educating their children at their best capacity. Whilst many would like for their children to receive an education, a large number of them do not want to take any risks in sending children to school as government promises do not stand for them. The aspirations after attainment of education are quite negligent among the family members of the Hadis and even among Bauris. Due to a lack of hope, education loses its importance in the eyes of the members of these communities. The data help to bring the stories of workplaces and the children of their employees and officers in the Steel Plant colony to light. The employed Hadis in steel plants refer to the place of work and aspire to create similar social conditions in the Hadi Cooli. However, nothing has been shared in terms of getting education and employment outside of this.

One person felt very proud when he introduced his two children to me during my fieldwork as a researcher. The reason was only that they were regularly going to school. This person is illiterate, but the kind of social interaction he has with other community members made him want to send (and impressed on him the importance of sending) his children to school. This person also has a television, which he got from his father-in-law. He watches programmes that are based on social issues, such as literacy missions and health-related campaigns with family members. The idea of a few parents to observe the everyday life of children is a bold step unlike many parents who have no time to monitor the educational and other everyday activities of their children. Those Hadi households make a point of making their home into a learning centre, and this is an important factor in the lives of poor Hadis; they consider it significant for their future endeavours. I tried to argue about the role of parents in the socialisation of children, which could be channelized, encouraged and adopted among the children, through different ways and modes of communication.

3. Aspects of Health Life in the Hadi Cooli

The health issue of Dalits has been discussed in the previous chapter. This chapter will focus on the basic health problems found among the Hadi caste. This is based on the data collected from the community during my fieldwork.

To fulfil the objectives of the present study, it is necessary to briefly describe the socio-economic condition of the Hadi community. This chapter gives a household profile of Hadis which helps us to locate the other issues related to their overall health.

To ensure *Health To All*, the Parliament of India approved a National Health Policy in 1983 as a common goal to be achieved by the then Government of India. This policy is meant to ensure that in health services provided by the state, major emphasis is placed on accessibility to the people; the availability of the infrastructure, social and cultural acceptability of the services, and affordability by lower socio-economic groups. The government of India has established several health centres but the proper functioning of these centres remains unquestioned. The number of health centres required across the region has not been reached; gross negligence towards the public health system has been a defining feature of the nation-state in India.

Table 3.1 Health Centres Established in India, 1995

Health Centres	Number of Health Centres
Sub-Centres	132,285
Primary Health Centres	21,802
Community Health Centres	2,401

There are many health centres which do not have any personal or technical health staff to handle the clinical and radiological cases. The absence of doctors is the most noticeable phenomenon hampering and minimising the usage of health care services. In light of this, these are some tables that show the empirical facts collected from and about the Hadi caste in the district of Bokaro.

Household Profiles: The profile of the study area has been discussed to look into the living conditions of the community. It will help to relate the socio-economic condition of the community to that of mainstream society.

Table 3.2 Household Profile of Hadis

Total H.H.	Total respondents			Total members			Sex Ratio	Total workers			Total literates		
38	T	M	F	T	M	F	F/100 M	T	M	F	T	M	F
	38	25	13	198	117	81	69	75	61	14	81	53	28

The above table (3.2) shows that the total number of respondents is 38, of which 25 are male and 13 are female. The total population is 198, of which 117 are male and 81 are female. The total working population is 75 in number, 61 being male and 14 being female. The total literate population is 81, comprising 53 males and only 28 females. The difference between male and female literacy is very high. Many female respondents were found to feel anger towards and anxiety within the social structure of Hindu caste-based society.

Early marriage is prevalent which adds to the vulnerability of women in this community. As they do not receive any formal education, they cannot access electronic and print media. This triple alliance of factors aggravates their situation. The process of socialisation within the households and outside the household of women plays a very crucial role. The overall personality of an individual reflects the kind of socialisation he or she gets.

The socialisation of young women and children within the house and family environment is more important than it is for men because women have less interaction with the outside world. Their behaviour and activities are always checked by neighbours, peers and general society in a case of gender bias. The table shows that fewer women are employed than are literate, but does not show that those who work are necessarily literate. Significantly it is reflected that women in sweeping caste groups have a higher share of percent in works except in the Hadi Cooli.

Age distribution of household members: Table 3.3 provides discussion which is very important for the understanding of the age distribution of the study population.

Table 3.3 Age distribution of household members

Total HH	10 and below		10-20		20-30		30-40		40-50		50 above	
38	M	F	M	F	M	F	M	F	M	F	M	F
	29	16	37	25	7	13	**12**	**13**	**18**	**13**	**4**	**1**
	45		**62**		**30**		**25**		**31**		**5**	

(Note: F- Female, M- Male)

Table 3.3 shows the age and sex distribution of household members. The total number of household sis 38. The number of male and female household members below age ten is 29 and16, respectively. Males between ten and twenty years of age number 37, compared with 25 female members for the same age group. The numbers of males and females between the age of twenty and thirty are 17 and 13 respectively. While there are 12 males and 13 females between thirty and forty, there are 18 males and 13 females between the ages of forty and fifty. Finally, those above fifty years of age make up a total of five: 4 males and 1 female respectively.

The highest number of individuals is found in the 10 to 20 age group, the second-largest number relates to members below the age of ten years, followed by 20 to 30 years of age.

Socio-Economic Characteristics of the study population: Socio-economic status is one determinant of the living condition of a population. The kind of employment available, and educational level (primary, secondary, or higher) are also important factors in deciding their status.

Table 3.4 Socio-economic characteristics

Sl. No.	Total workers			Total literates		
1	T	M	F	T	M	F
2	**75**	**61**	**14**	**81**	**53**	**28**

The above table (3.4) shows the socio-economic characteristics of the respondents including individuals of *Hadi* caste. The ratio of working to total population may vary if we compare it with other caste groups; however, this table provides a background to explore overall work status.

Among a total of 75 working individuals, 61 males are found to be working, whatever the type of work, compared with only 14 female individuals. This table does not give details of occupational categories, which have been included in a separate table later on in the chapter.

The rate of unemployment has not reduced despite the fact that the district has a good number of industries. Even Bokaro Steel Plant has not been helpful in decreasing unemployment among Dalits unlike many other castes groups who have found employment. There are several coal reserve areas as one of the main strengths of the district Bokaro is coal mining. For instance, Bermo-sub division of Bokaro district comprises few coal mining sites and huge coal reserves. But the job employability of Dalits is quite negligible as reported by the people who work in these coal mines.

Table 3.5 Total Family Incomes (Yearly)

Respondent	**Total Family Income (annually)**				**Total**
	<10	10-20	20-30	30>	
Male	14	9	1	1	25
Female	12	1	0	0	13
Total	**36**	**10**	**1**	**1**	**38**

This table (3.5) shows the yearly income of households as reported by the respondents. To understand and present this in a simple way, income has been divided into four categories. These four income classifications represent the economic background of each household interviewed. The four categories are divided as: income below 10,000 rupees per year, income between 10 to 20,000 rupees per year, income between 20 to 30,000 rupees per year and income above 30,000 rupees per year.

Most of the respondents (26), 14 men and 12 women, earn less than 10,000 rupees annually. The annual income ranges between 10,000-20,000 for ten respondents, out of which nine are men. One male respondent falls in the twenty to thirty thousand category and another earns above thirty thousand but no female individuals fall in either two categories. Twelve women out of a total of thirteen earn less than 10,000 thousand rupees; only one belongs to the second category, earning between 10,000-20,000 thousand. If we combine male and female income into a single category, 68 percent fall in the lowest income group, of earning below 10,000 rupees. Twenty six percent fall in the second category and three percent each are in the other two categories.

Besides economic prosperity, availability of health care services and willingness to utilise them are important. It is established in earlier studies that utilization of health care services not only depends on availability of health care centres, but social and cultural barrier also need to be curtailed.

As part of total health care, issues related to family planning material, child health, and immunisation have been examined. Family planning services are availed by 13 respondents, out of them 11 are men and 2 are women. Awareness regarding the services and availability of the services both appeared to be poor. The qualitative data illustrates that social interaction between Hadis (Dalit among Dalits) have almost invisible contact over the matters of community life. The government officials and health staffs do not enter into the Hadi Cooli. There have been several occasions when a health worker collects the health profile from outsiders or anyone caught outside the Hadi Cooli, as houses are close together.

House Ownership and Type: Housing has a crucial role to play in the living conditions of human beings. A welfare state such as India is supposed to provide basic amenities and all other facilities to every citizen especially to the marginalized Dalits as Hadis. This has been examined on the basis of table 3.6 below.

Table 3.6 House Type and House Ownership

House Type	House Ownership		Total
	Rented	Owned	
Kutcha	1	34	25
Semi Pucca	0	3	3
	1	37	38

The above table shows the pattern of house ownership. Most of the respondents (37) had their own houses. Only one respondent lived in a rented house, which was a Kutcha house. Among those who owned their house, 34 lived in kutcha and 3 in semi-pucca houses. This data shows that house ownership is quite high. The congested and crowded housing condition is one of the factors which has some relationship to the overall health of the community. The health of people is grossly affected by the kind of house they have and reside into. The following table shows the number of house and type of house.

Table 3.7 House Type and Number of Rooms

House Type	Number of Rooms			Total
	1	2	3	
Kutcha	11	23	1	35
Semi Pucca	0	1	2	3
Total	11	24	3	38

The above table shows the distribution by the number of rooms per household. Out of the 35 respondents who lived in kutcha houses, 11 had one-room units, 23 had two-room units and 1 had a three-room unit. For those who lived in semi-pucca houses, 1 household had a two-room unit and 2 had three-room units. The number of semi-pucca owning households is the lowest. Only 3 respondents reported having a semi-pucca house. Among them, 1 household had two rooms and 2 had two rooms.

Housing conditions are very poor among this community. Housing is an important factor affecting individual health. If we divide the number of household members per room this results as 5.21 per room; this is a very high ratio of person to room which shows restricted and congested living conditions. Park and Park (1991), state that "housing not only includes the 'physical structure' providing shelter, but also the immediate surroundings, and the related community services and facilities" (pp.394). The World Health Organisation (WHO) has also given its own term "residential environment" which is defined as the "physical structure that man uses and the environs of that structure including all necessary services, facilities, equipment and devices needed or desired for the physical and mental health and social well-being of the family and the individual" (Park and Park, 1991, 394-395).

1. To put it briefly, a healthy residential environment is one in which "the family can develop and flourish physically, mentally and socially".
2. The immediate surroundings of residential buildings are often referred to as the neighbourhood or micro-district. (Park and Park, 395).

The Hadi Cooli is only a small area of land. An expert committee of the WHO recommended the following criteria for healthful housing similar to the "Basic Principles of Healthful Housing" paper published by the American Public Health Association (APA).

1. Healthful housing provides physical protection and shelter,
2. Provides adequately for cooking, eating, washing and excretory functions,
3. Is designed, constructed, maintained and used in a manner such as to prevent the spread of communicable diseases,
4. Provides for protection from hazards of exposure to noise and pollution,
5. Is free from unsafe physical arrangements due to construction or maintenance, and from toxic or harmful materials, and
6. Encourages personal and community development promotes social relationships, reflects a regard for ecological principals, and by these means promotes mental health.

A majority of households do not have space for cooking within the premises of their house. This adds to the vulnerability of the housing condition of this vulnerable section of the population. The social surroundings of urban society are very distinct from the rural set up. There is a great pain to any researcher to understand that the problem of the urban settlements belonging to urban society is very distinct from the urban settlements belonging to underprivileged groups. *Hadis* desire to buy new land at other sites of the township. Inequality among this community is increasing in comparison to mainstream society. Their income has not increased for the last ten years, whereas the market situation has become dynamic. The increasing cost of everyday items has negative consequences. They cannot buy more than food, for everyday or other purposes.

Overcrowding is increasing with the growth of the population. New data emerges in Bokaro showing the level of migration to other places. Not even a single household of the settlement of Dalits (studied population) has migrated to another city, except for relocation to nearby localities within the Bokaro. Housing and health are strongly interlinked because there are factors like pollution and hazards of the menial occupation in sweeping, and cleaning toilets. The occupation of cleaning filthy toilets and public drains without proper safety equipment and measures when required, apart from during the removal of the blockage of the drains, tends to be the responsible factor for the decline in health. Some diseases such as respiratory and skin infections are found in higher ratios in overcrowded houses, and the rates of mortality and morbidity are high where housing conditions are sub-standard. This is why there is a standard defining an acceptable ratio of room/person. Parks and Parks (1991) elaborate these understandings as follows:

One room can accommodate only two persons and two rooms can hold three persons etc. but this standardized criteria to understand the Dalits of Hadis is neither possible to apply nor feasible to expect in the studied community. There is an urgent need to increase the proportion of rooms per individual. This is only possible when their socio-economic condition is improved. The sources of their livelihood will be siphoned away, once the election for the local governing bodies is done. These people have to be accommodated in the vacant opportunities in employment.

Table 3.8 House Type and Drainage

House type	Drains			Total
	Open	None	Any other	
Kutcha	16	17	2	35
Semi-Pucca	2	1	-	3
Total	18	18	2	38

Note: "any other" refers those who have dug a ditch for disposed water.

Table 3.8 reports on house type and drains and gives an idea of the drainage condition in the Hadi Cooli. Out of thirty-eight households, eighteen had an open drain and eighteen had no drain, thus no cutlet for used water. There were two households who reported drying the gravel to release used water underneath earth. Once the ditch is full, it is covered with mud. In the need of water for domestic purposes, people use various traditional techniques to fetch water. In the last twenty years of time, Chas town has witnessed depleting underground water. Municipal corporation (Nagarpalika) has failed to provide the tap water and it has again been made part of the 2027 AD Chas Municipal Planning Document.

House type distribution by drainage systems is shown in table 2. Out of 35 respondents who live in kutcha houses, 16 have open drains, 17 had no drains and the rest did not have a bath. They dispose of waste water in the ditch. 2 households had open drains and 1 household had no drain at all.

The Hadi Cooli has no proper drainage system, which is evident from this table. The whole area surrounding the settlement has no or only partial drainage during the fieldwork conducted for the present study. There has been no election in the state until 2010 for local governing bodies for more than two decades.

During the monsoon, there is water logging in front of the Hadi Cooli. Other areas are better off in terms of drainage. Residents also need to maintain cleanliness by not throwing the garbage into the drain and allowing it to clog. They often use their hands to clear clogged drains.

Source of Drinking Water: The basic need of the community as regards drinking water is not fulfilled. Each family has to walk a long distance to fetch water for drinking. This is one distinct feature of the indignity and crisis Hadis have now faced for decades. Since the separation of the Bokaro district from the Dhanbad district, it has never improved.

Table 3.9 Drinking Water: Sources and Consumption

Source of drinking water	**Public tap**	**Well**		**Hand Pump**			**Total**	
No. of H.H.	32	4		2			38	
Consumption of water (buckets per day)								
Buckets	<5	**6-10 Buckets**					10>	
		6	7	8	9	10		
No. of H.H.	2	7	2	18	3	4	1	1

***H.H. – Household**

Drinking water availability is a significant problem in these areas. The above tables show that water is available to the households of all the respondents either through a public tap or from a well. No one in the community has access to drinking water in the "Mohalla". However, thirty-two respondents reported that their source of drinking water is the public tap, which is about one kilometre away. Five households have access to the well. The well they use belongs to the Shakara caste but is not permissible for everyone. This drinking well belongs to the individual family, therefore, not regularly. One single-hand pump is located in the centre of the Shakara Cooli on the temple's premises. Hadis are not allowed here. The rest of the Bauri castes reportedly used the source at the temple premise, but Hadis used a public tap near Mahabir Chowk, Chas. Other sources refer to the mixed or multiple-use responses comprising hand pumps mostly and the well or public tap occasionally. There are a few hand pumps located at the nearest market, one inside the premise of Chas police station, which is rarely used by this community. These people do not have clean or hygienic drinking water sources where they can bathe and wash clothes. Untouchability is a part of their socio-cultural and political life. This creates a continuous chain of discrimination towards Dalits who experience the non-availability of basic needs and amenities in the community area.

Early in the morning, a long queue for fetching water is part of the daily routine. Women and young girls have the main responsibility for these jobs. One needs to figure out the quality of the water. This doubt arises from the fact that the location of the water tap is just at the upper side of the *Joria* (i.e. "*Nala*" or drain, which takes the form of a stream of wastewater).

The understanding of the interplay and integration of two ecological universes determine the health status of an individual, a community or a nation: the internal environment of man and the external environment, which surround him. In the modern concept, "disease is due to a disturbance in the delicate balance between man and his environment" (Park and Park 1991, 367).

Drinking water is used only for domestic purposes such as drinking, cooking, or washing utensils or pots. Talking about safe drinking water seems a matter only for policymakers; reality tells a very different story. Not a single individual in the Hadi community knows that safe water should be free from pathogenic agents; free from harmful chemical substances; pleasant to the taste; and not preferred for domestic purposes. Providing clean water to this community at the doorstep (of every household) is urgent. The Municipal Corporation, on the practical level, does not exist in this area. This means there is no way of providing water for domestic purposes at the settlement itself.

Another important factor to consider in the context of the availability of safe and clean water is the duration of the tapped water's availability and the consumption volume. Regarding duration, the supply is more or less once in twenty-four hours. The consumption of water is evident from the above table. Table 3.9 (see above) shows the daily consumption of water for domestic purposes, i.e. water requirement for drinking, cooking, bathing and washing. The table shows the classification of the respondents' responses according to water use per day. Most respondents are seen in the eight buckets per day (one bucket is used as a unit to represent an average capacity size of around 20 litres of water). It is based on the general understanding of fellow community members in terms of the approximate number of buckets they fill. Eighteen respondents said they used eight buckets per day. Seven respondents use ten buckets, and seven use six buckets per day. Two households consume seven buckets per day. In the above cases, the use of water for domestic purposes does not include water used for bathing and washing. These two activities are undertaken at the nearest pond, which is very dirty.

To Dalits in Chas, the theoretical or hygienic definition of clean water differs in their place, and the first and foremost point that appears essential is that water is available at any source. Later the hygiene and cleanliness of water are discussed. Their socio-economic condition does not allow them to dig a well or set up a hand pump. It costs thousands to install and have such a thing at one's capacity. Socially neglected sections of the past and present population of Dalits as Hadis are side-lined in all spheres of life. Although one may not see any significant change in the political or economic fields, they are given some social space in mainstream society. The Hadi community, settled in the centre of the town and serving, for the most part, the city's invaluable and necessary cleaning activity, needs proper access to the basic requirements of life. These sentences are repetitive; remove the first, starting with "Two major sources."

Table 3.10 Electricity: Duration of Power Supply

Electricity	**Duration of power supply (hours per day)**					**Total**
	12	**16**	**18**	**20**	**NA**	
Yes	1	8	21	5	0	**35**
No	0	0	0	0	3	**3**
Total	1	8	21	5	3	**3**

Note: N.A means "Not Available".

The above table (3.10) shows the differences in duration of the power supply in this area. Jharkhand is among the highest power generation states in the country, yet the power conditions are also the most pathetic in terms of its availability to the poorest of the state. The largest chunk of the power supply is given and sold to other states including the national capital, Delhi. Out of 35 households in the study, three do not have electricity. Among those who do, twenty-one (21) reported to have eighteen hours of power followed by eight who only have power supply for sixteen hours. Five households had a supply for twenty hours. Only one household is reported to have twelve hours of power supply.

The above scenario does not accurately represent the overall condition of apathy and deprivation that the Hadi caste faces in their everyday lives. For instance, if there is a fault with the electric supplying wire, it takes weeks to get it reported to the department concerned. There are a few pockets in Chas where every household has an electric supply connection but electricity is rarely found. Local community members do make efforts at times in the direction of getting a regular power supply but generally in vain.

Hadis are economically very weak and thus cannot afford the burden of repair costs, such as calling an electrician and offering him some wages. So most of the time they either try to resolve the problem themselves or have to wait for the electricity staff to conduct repair work voluntarily.

However, as reported by the respondents, the power situation has slightly improved, in comparison to earlier years. Most Dalit houses have electricity connection in any form but the supply is quite low. The reason given is the division of the state from erstwhile Bihar in November of the year 2000. This perception was enforced during the Focus Group Discussion (FGD) about the power station with the Bauri caste. Bauri caste families, too, face continuous deprivation and negligence by the governmental machineries and administrative authority of the municipal corporation.

Concluding Observations

The socio-demographic (household) profile of the people who participated in the study is the primary emphasis of this chapter. The household profile shows that the women, in particular, have a relatively low level of literacy, which indicates the low level of social position of Hadi women. The level of education in a community is a vital measure of the social life that exists there. Hadis demonstrates that out of a total of 160 members of a family, there are 55 who are illiterate. On the other hand, other groups of people have either completed basic school or are pursuing their education. There is a direct correlation between the total income of a family and the educational level of its members since these cash-enabled families send their children to school, at the very least through elementary school. The housing situation in the community is a reflection of the interplay of all of the elements listed above. Concerning the number of people living in a given space, not a single respondent has a pucca home, and only three of them have semi-pucca dwellings. Given the low levels of income, the desire to own a pucca house that has more than two rooms remains a faraway goal for many people, even if there are many people who actually own their own house. The additional space has the potential to be roomier and less crowded. The age of the drains and the source of the water are two of the most important factors to consider when evaluating the health of any community, and the fact that Hadis in Chas are among the most discriminated Dalits demonstrates that these factors have a severe influence on their health. The absence of publicly supported infrastructure contributes to already deplorable living conditions. Electricity, which is a necessary component of city life, is accessible to them, and this may be interpreted as a good aspect of their way of life. In conclusion, the profile that was created here reveals that the socio-economic position of Hadis is not at all adequate, and their general morbidity pattern reflects the need for health care facilities. This need was reflected in the fact that they had a need for health care facilities.

CHAPTER FOUR

LINKAGES BETWEEN HEALTH AND SOCIAL EXCLUSION AMONG HADIS – THE AXES OF DENIAL

Introduction

The concept of "health" is quite multifaceted and may be used in a variety of settings. Therefore, the meanings of health and people's perceptions of their health are not the same. Various academics and professionals in the field of public health have provided colourful definitions of the term "health." "Health is not simply the absence of disease," according to the official definition of "health" that was established by the World Health Organisation (WHO) in 1974. This definition states that "health is the rate of complete physical, mental, spiritual, and social well-being." Jones asserts that people's perceptions "about health and morbidity are connected to wider social, cultural, and material factors" (Jones 1994). He cites this assertion in his work. The question of how to describe an individual's state of health has always been contentious.

It has always been difficult to agree on how to characterise an individual's state of health. This issue could be mitigated by "presenting its socio-economic indicators, rate of population increase, per capita GNP, level of unemployment, dependency ratio, literacy rates, and especially female literacy rates, family size, persons living in one room, per capita 'caloric' availability, excluding other indicators" (Park and Park 1991). These are some of the indicators that make up socio-economic indicators. Other indicators include the availability of other indicators.

In a similar vein, the problem of defining morbidity is a difficult one to solve. It is self-evident that it plays a vital role and is a major factor in determining the health status of a community or nation. Morbidity may be an indicator of any particular population's health state and the risk associated with sickness; however, it is not an accuracy measure. The state of being unwell, disabled, or afflicted with an ailment is referred to as morbidity. The rates of morbidity, the frequency of morbidity, the length of morbidity, and the severity of morbidity are the three additional elements of morbidity that are employed for measurement. The mortality rate, on the other hand, does not accurately reflect the situation at any given moment; rather, it obscures the true picture. In spite of the fact that the crude death rate does not give precision since it does not take into account the age disparities in age structure, it is a well-known fact that the number of deaths per 1,000 persons in the midyear population However, this statistic might be misleading when making comparisons.

The purpose of this chapter is to make an attempt to talk about and think about the issues surrounding morbidity in Hadi Cooli and how they impact the lives of the members of families there. Therefore, in order to evaluate the morbidity pattern of the community in Hadi Cooli, existing empirical data are employed to contextualise the concerns. The pattern of morbidity illustrates the state of the Dalits' health in Chas in the field region. Chas is still a very significant town, and its lengthy history of human habitation dates back to the time when West Bengal was still dominated by the British empire. The table that follows demonstrates an intriguing insight and helps study how an occupational group of manual scavengers carry out their day-to-day activities while having a debilitating health condition.

Reported Morbidity Pattern

Table 5.1 Morbidity among Respondents

Disease	**Male**	**Female**	**Total**
Tuberculosis (T.B)	6	4	**10**
Skin Diseases/infections	7	5	12
Low Blood Pressure	1	1	2
Gynaecological Problems	0	10	10
Eye Sight	1	1	2
Chest pain	1	1	2
Asthma	3	0	3
Long Term Ailments	**19**	**22**	**41**
Weakness	4	7	11
Headache	11	7	18
Body-ache	14	11	25
Backache	13	9	22
Fever	23	13	36
Cold and cough	21	12	33

General Recurring	**86**	**59**	**145**
Jaundice	2	0	2
Malaria	6	4	10
Diarrhoea	4	3	7
Chickenpox	1	0	1
Short Term Ailments	13	7	20
Grand Total	**118**	**58**	**206**

The total number of respondents who reported having negative health experiences is presented in the table above. On the basis of the data shown in Table 1, the respondents' illnesses have been divided into three categories: conditions that last for a long time, conditions that last for a short time, and general recurrent illnesses. Table 1 displays the mortality rates experienced by residents of the area under investigation. The majority of respondents (145) reported suffering from general illnesses, followed by short-term/episodic (42) and long-term (10) complaints. The majority of them (69) reported having fever, cough, and cold symptoms. A total of 25 of the respondents reported having body aches, followed by backaches (22) and headaches (18).

There were a total of thirty-eight (38) people who participated in the survey; 25 of them were male and 13 of them were female. There is one table for male respondents and one table for female respondents that each indicate their respective occupations and morbidities. There are six different types of occupations that have been created based on the responses of the respondents. The men are responsible for the hard tasks, which include sweeping, rickshaw pulling, and garbage collection by hand. On the other hand, the majority of the responders who are female are involved in activities such as sweeping, scavenging, and household work. Dais are a traditional birth attendant who has been assisting community members with all aspects of pregnancy and childbirth for many years.

The morbidity among respondents has been classified by the use of classification. In comparison to the other villages, this one has a significantly greater prevalence of illness. A poor diet can lead to malnutrition, which is especially prevalent in young children and women. It is difficult for the primary health centres (PHCs) in Chas to capture and keep records on patients' health trends, as well as their use of health services and other related topics. When the chief medical officer (CMO) of the Primary Health Centre (PHC) neglected to provide details of the couples who had availed themselves of family planning services or of those who were suffering from disease, the justification given was that the carelessness was due to the fact that involved departments had provided insufficient funds. Despite this, a few employees asserted that “sanitation has improved since the state of Jharkhand separated from the former state of Bihar.”

Although there is a lack of governmental commitment to primary health care in India, the initial theoretical focus of PHC has been quite strong. When it comes to providing the most convenient access to medical care, the participation of local governing bodies is absolutely necessary. This action will raise the likelihood that the disadvantaged will see an improvement in their current state of health.

“Equity in health care, need-based; socially acceptable service with full participation of peoples’ state responsibility for incorporating PHCs into national development plans through inter-sectoral strategies; affordable technologies ensuring self-sufficiency and effective basic health care with the support of secondary and tertiary care; and collective, net individual efforts” is what Qadeer (2001, 118–19) identifies as the fundamental importance of primary health care centres. Additionally, underrepresented groups within the population need to be educated on both their rights and responsibilities. It is not true that there is no provision for the provision of fundamental services in the field of health care. However, neither the availability nor the accessibility of services to individuals who have a need for them are guaranteed in any way.

During my meeting with the director of the district hospitals, I had the opportunity to speak with Dr. Jairam, the civil surgeon. He informed me that “Bokaro is one of the most highly endemic Malaria zones.” A distance of many kilometres separates you from the district sub-divisional hospital that serves the area. Members of the Hadi caste are prevented from accessing the offered facilities due to a number of circumstances, not the least of which is the location and distance of the hospital. In addition, a persistent stereotypical image of public health institutions has been tremendously detrimental to the populations that reside there. This image is defined by ignorance, unpleasant attitudes of the health employees and physicians, the non-availability of medications, and doctors’ irregular attendance in the hospitals and health facilities where they are needed. Hadis asserts that physicians have a discriminatory attitude towards lower-income and more “degraded” areas.

When researchers went to the several health centres in question, they found that these variables were enhanced. To be of assistance to the current study, it was necessary to get certain basic and general data; however, the information could not be obtained due to the presence of a great number of unspecified causes. In fact, looking for this information consumed a significant amount of time and effort over the course of two months. Ironically, the researchers were only successful in obtaining the information after making contact with the Deputy Commissioner (DC) of the Bokaro region.

It would appear that the most difficult goal for Hadis to accomplish is to have access to the health care services offered by PHCs. As long as there is not a significant shift in the whole social hierarchy that is present in the organisation of the health care sector, the concept of the state's obligation to give "health to all" will continue to be a nightmare. The Bhore Committee (1946), also known as the Health Survey and Development Committee, had suggested the outlawing of private practise by public doctors; however, this recommendation is not implemented at every level of the design and implementation of health care. Sir Joseph Bhore served as the chairman of the Bhore Committee. The social exclusion of lower caste groups is systematically influenced by caste dynamics. During the course of the research, an interview was conducted with the district civil surgeon, who is a member of a lower caste group. At that time, he expressed a great deal of displeasure when the researcher made notes on information and interaction about the indifference of the district health administration towards Dalits. He did not give off the impression of being pleased or at ease with the attitudes of his fellow physicians and other colleagues. Throughout the course of the interview with the surgeon, other doctors were actively participating and making repeated attempts to steer the conversation in a direction that was not pertinent to the goals of the research. They were upsetting and attempted to persuade the researcher that this sort of research does not benefit those who have been ostracised from society. It was made very apparent that Dalits, also known as Hadis, do not merit any assistance or incentives; rather, they are the ones who are accountable for their own fate and destiny.

The morbidity rate for the respondents is presented in Table 1. In total, there are three categories of illness that may be distinguished from one another. This is further extended based on the International Disease Classification (IDC), which categorises diseases throughout the world. However, this categorization does not adequately meet our requirements because the IDC does not account for all of the disorders that are presented in the table.

Health can be defined as "the rate of complete physical, mental, spiritual, and social well-being." Jones asserts that people's perceptions "about health and morbidity are connected to wider social, cultural, and material factors" (Jones 1994). He cites this assertion in his work. The question of how to describe an individual's state of health has always been contentious.

It has always been difficult to agree on how to characterise an individual's state of health. This issue could be mitigated by "presenting its socio-economic indicators, rate of population increase, per capita GNP, level of unemployment, dependency ratio, literacy rates, and especially female literacy rates, family size, persons living in one room, per capita 'caloric' availability, excluding other indicators" (Park and Park 1991). These are some of the indicators that make up socio-economic indicators. Other indicators include the availability of other indicators.

In a similar vein, the problem of defining morbidity is a difficult one to solve. It is self-evident that it plays a vital role and is a major factor in determining the health status of a community or nation. Morbidity may be an indicator of any particular population's health state and the risk associated with sickness; however, it is not an accuracy measure. The state of being unwell, disabled, or afflicted with an ailment is referred to as morbidity. The rates of morbidity, the frequency of morbidity, the length of morbidity, and the severity of morbidity are the three additional elements of morbidity that are employed for measurement. The mortality rate, on the other hand, does not accurately reflect the situation at any given moment; rather, it obscures the true picture. In spite of the fact that the crude death rate does not give precision since it does not take into account the age disparities in age structure, it is a well-known fact that the number of deaths per 1,000 persons in the midyear population However, this statistic might be misleading when making comparisons.

The purpose of this chapter is to make an attempt to talk about and think about the issues surrounding morbidity in Hadi Cooli and how they impact the lives of the members of families there. Therefore, in order to evaluate the morbidity pattern of the community in Hadi Cooli, existing empirical data are employed to contextualise the concerns. The pattern of morbidity illustrates the state of the Dalits' health in Chas in the field region. Chas is still a very significant town, and its lengthy history of human habitation dates back to the time when West Bengal was still dominated by the British empire. The table that follows demonstrates an intriguing insight and helps study how an occupational group of manual scavengers carry out their day-to-day activities while having a debilitating health condition.

Respiratory Infection

Due to the settings in which they work and their possible exposure to both illnesses, those who engage in menial and dirty jobs are more vulnerable to both chickenpox and TB.

The varicella-zoster virus, which causes chickenpox, is a very infectious virus. The danger of infection spreading is higher in soiled and grubby jobs when workers are in close proximity to one another and hygiene standards may be breached. The following are some effects of chickenpox on those who work in certain fields:

Chickenpox can be contracted through direct contact with the fluid from an infected person's blisters or by respiratory droplets. The virus may spread quickly from one person to another in crowded, filthy workplaces, which can cause outbreaks among employees. Absence from Work: Although chickenpox often resolves on its own, it can still result in severe pain, fever, and skin rashes. If affected people do not have access to paid sick leave, they may need to take time out of work to recuperate, which might result in lost productivity and financial burden. Although uncommon, the consequences of chickenpox can be severe, particularly in adults and those with compromised immune systems. Due to the nature of their work environment, employees in menial and dirty industries may be more likely to experience difficulties if they develop chickenpox.

Mycobacterium tuberculosis is the bacterium that causes the disease TB. Although it mostly affects the lungs, it can extend to other body areas. The following variables may increase the risk of TB among workers in shabby and unclean occupations:

Congested areas with inadequate ventilation: When a person with tuberculosis coughs or sneezes, it spreads via the air. The bacterium may quickly transfer from one person to another in crowded and poorly ventilated environments. Weakening of Immune Systems: Workers' immune systems may get weakened as a result of working in unsanitary settings and being exposed to other illnesses, leaving them more vulnerable to contracting TB infections.

Delayed Diagnosis and Treatment: Due to a variety of factors, such as financial restrictions or a lack of knowledge, employees in soiled and menial jobs may have restricted access to healthcare services and may choose to ignore early TB symptoms. The danger of spreading TB to others rises with delayed diagnosis and treatment, which can result in more severe forms of the disease.

Nutrition and health: People who work in these jobs are more susceptible to TB and its sequelae because of poor nutrition and living circumstances, which can further degrade their health.

Therefore, both chicken pox and TB can have a significant negative impact on the health and productivity of people who perform menial and dirty work. In order to lessen the occurrence of these illnesses and their effects on vulnerable groups, it is crucial to improve cleanliness, provide access to treatment, and raise knowledge about them.

In the field data, tuberculosis and chickenpox are the two respiratory diseases reported by respondents. A total of six cases of TB were found among males and four among female respondents. A specific infection of TB disease is caused by mycobacterium tuberculosis that spreads in a person's body in the lungs when coughs or sneezes. The active TB disease in a human puts out the bacteria and the same is inhaled by others nearby to the bacteria, get TB. The disease primarily effects lungs and causes pulmonary tuberculosis. Pulmonary tuberculosis is the most important form of TB found among men. However, it was not clear from the responses to which group of disease respondents belonged; they have not properly been treated for TB at the public health centre.

Table 5.2 Morbidity by Occupation and Disease (Male)

Occupation / Disease	Scavenging	Sweeper	Rickshaw-puller	Manual Labour	Total
TB	2	2	1	1	**6**
Malaria	1	1	3	1	**6**
Asthma	1	1	1	0	**3**
Cold and Cough	7	9	3	2	**21**
Fever	11	5	2	5	**23**
Skin Disease	4	2	0	1	**7**
Weakness	2	1	1	0	**4**
Headache	5	3	2	1	**11**
Total	33	24	13	11	**81**

Note: Table 5.2 does not include all diseases.

Out of the total of thirty-eight respondents, including male and female respondents, the bad health experiences of twenty-five male respondents are shown in the above table (5.2), which is based on the reported illness pattern. An interview was conducted with one person from each home, and questions centred on diseases experienced in the previous six months. The table displays the illness distribution by profession for a specific disease across many occupations. The purpose is to emphasise each person's employment and state of health.

Twenty-five (25) male respondents made up the sample, and they worked as rickshaw pullers, scavengers, sweepers, and other manual labourers. Understanding the morbidity and employment of respondents is made easier by this categorization. There were six documented TB cases, which were further broken down based on occupational bifurcation. Two guys were discovered working as scavengers out of the total of six instances, while the other two were discovered sweeping. One person pulled rickshaws (01) and another (01) did physical tasks.

The manual scavengers, or Hadis, are typically required to labour whenever families need assistance. Sometimes Hadis transport night-soil from clogged toilet drains, although this has decreased as more people are turning to septic tanks and changing the types of toilets. They are unable to grow up in a clean environment. Along with performing laborious and menial work, inadequate nutrition and congestion make life more difficult. There's no need to mention that as people age, their immune systems weaken. In this population, there is a higher risk of infection.

Because they only seek treatment at medical facilities for significant health conditions, respondents could only describe the symptoms of the ailments they had. Six (6) cases of malarial encounters were discovered in total. Three instances among rickshaw drivers were recorded, then one case each in the categories of scavenging, sweeping, and manual labour. With the exception of the manual labour category, each group reported one incidence of asthma, totaling three (3) instances.

However, among the twenty-one (21) instances of cold and cough, sweepers had the largest number (nine), followed by scavengers with seven cases. Only three instances among rickshaw drivers and two among manual labourers were documented. There were seven skin disease cases documented. Scavengers accounted for four of them, followed by sweepers with two and manual labourers with one. Rickshaw pullers did not have a single instance documented. The first three groups were the only ones to exhibit weakness. There are several incidences of headaches, including five in the first group of scavengers, three among sweepers, two among rickshaw pullers, and one among the manual labourers.

Table 5.3 Morbidity by Occupation (Female)

Occupation Disease	Scavenging	Sweeping	*Dai*	Domestic work	Total
TB	2	1	1	0	4
Malaria	1	2	0	1	4
Asthma	0	0	0	0	0
Cold and Cough	3	7	1	1	12
Fever	3	3	4	3	13
Skin Disease	2	1	2	0	5
Weaknesses	1	1	2	3	7
Headache	1	2	1	3	7
Gynaecological Problems	2	5	0	3	10
Body-ache	5	4	0	2	11
Total	20	26	11	16	73

Note: table 5.3 shows the illness suffered by female respondents working in different occupations

There are nearly as many women as men in the world's population. The interview took place in Hadi Cooli, which is a tiny hamlet that is primarily involved in the manual scavenging vocation and has been accorded a certain social standing as a result. Not only does an individual's socioeconomic and political environment reflect their social rank, but so does the power that is associated with that level. This also includes political standing, which is relevant in cases where the economy plays a significant role in a specific society, such as in Chas town. The lack of an economic foundation and organisation among Dalits (also known as Hadis) contributes to overall poor conditions. The powerful force of change that is impacting the Dalits in India is similarly affecting the Hadi community. This is proved by the truth that cultural lag is a continual process of all the social groupings and communities that exist at the current time. The material culture of the location and the city has not had a substantial effect on the lives of Hadis, and it has left behind the tradition of continuing family and caste jobs. A decline in one's health, whether it be physical, mental, or psychological, can be brought on by a number of different factors.

If we look at Table 5.3, we can see that the percentage of respondents who suffer from disease is not minor at all. According to this number, the rate of sickness sustained by female respondents is not lower than that of male respondents. The disparity may be attributed to the fact that out of a total of 38 respondents, only 13 of them are women, which accounts for 34 percent of the total.

Scavenging, sweeping, housekeeping, and Da'i (Birth Attendant) are some of the occupations that are grouped together under the umbrella of the female respondents' four larger occupational categories. There are a total of four (4) female responders who have been diagnosed with tuberculosis. Of these four, two are involved in scavenging, and the other two are involved in sweeping and Dai work, respectively. Malaria is reported to be prevalent in this part of the world. Malaria-causing mosquitoes thrive in environments that are conducive to their development, such as open drains that are clogged with debris and standing water in drains. People who suffer from fever quite frequently are unaware of the specific form of fever that they have. The chart demonstrates an increase in the number of patients suffering from malaria.

Out of the 12 instances of cold and cough, 25% of the females were engaged in scavenging, while 7 responded that they were engaged in sweeping. There was only one case in each of the groups engaged in employment as a domestic helper or as a Dai. There have been reports of three cases of fever among female scavengers and another three cases among those working as sweepers. On the other hand, respondents have reported four cases of fever among the Dai, and the remaining three cases are identified among domestic employees. Scavengers were responsible for two of the five cases of skin illness that were discovered, and another two cases were discovered between Dais. The sweeping category was responsible for the last case. Three of the seven (7) people who were ill with weakness had been doing household labour; two had been acting as Dai; and one had been doing both sweeping and scavenging, respectively.

There was a total of ten (10) cases of gynaecological issues that were recorded, two of which were found to be the result of scavenging, five of which were the result of sweeping, and three of which were connected to working on domestic tasks. 11 of the total 13 respondents reported having body aches, with five from the group that scavenged, four from the group that swept, and two from the group that did domestic labour reporting having body aches. There was no indication that any of them suffered from asthma, and the female respondents were unable to recall any additional difficulties they had experienced in the preceding half year. The health of Dalit women who belong to the Hadi caste is in very poor condition. They are required to work not only in their own homes but also in the homes of other people in order to contribute financially to the family. Their lives are made more difficult than those of any other socioeconomic group in that region as a result of this double load, in particular for Hadi women, who have greater rates of anaemia.

The deteriorating state of this group's health must be understood in the context of their socio-economic standing in order to be fully comprehended. The vast majority of the overall workforce is rendered unable to function. The number of people in the caste group who are dependent on others, namely children, is growing. There are not enough vacant positions for women in the workforce. It is forbidden for women to leave their cramped homes, and they must remain there in order to complete their domestic responsibilities. In accordance with their customs and rituals, they are not required to live in such deplorable circumstances; instead, they are required to spend the majority of their time in a cramped ghetto and a filthy street, oftentimes right next to open drains. On the other hand, those who belong to lower castes have a lower social standing, while those who belong to higher castes have a greater social status. This is true in the field. However, during the group discussion with older women and men, it was found that women who participated in household tasks had a greater degree of independence in their day-to-day lives than women who belonged to other higher social castes in the area. In contrast to some of Chas's higher castes, Chas's society as a whole does not practise overt gender discrimination. The patriarchy has historically been compelled to acknowledge the necessity of women's domestic labour by the coercive forces of great deprivation and marginalisation. Women in Hadi culture are treated with the respect and importance that are due to them by both the general populace and the elders. This is seen in the manner in which food is provided during marriage ceremonies for members of the Hadi caste. On the occasion of any marriage among the Hadis, the meal is served starting with the women and children, then moving on to the senior members, and finally moving on to the other members.

Table 5.4 Utilisation of Family Planning Services

Serial No.	Respondents	Family Planning Services Availed		Total
		Yes	No	
1	Male	11	14	25
2	Female	2	11	13
	Total	13	25	38

Note: this table 5.4 shows the responses of respondents who have availed any FP services.

The provision of both permanent and temporary methods of contraception is included in the services offered by family planning organisations. The vast majority of the respondents had utilised contraceptive pills or other preventative techniques indicated by the local RMPs. Occasionally, Auxiliary Nurse Midwives (ANM) had also induced women to carry home contraceptives tablets whenever they visited PHCs. There is minimal prejudice in promoting family planning techniques because every primary health care provider and staff member gets a flash marked excellent comment from the higher authorities for achieving the highest objectives in family planning. Free condoms are offered to interested spouses, and there is minimal discrimination.

Services relating to family planning are included in the medical treatment that people get. Despite this, the plan is unable to achieve its primary goals as a result of a number of obstacles that are of a political, geographical, and socio-cultural character. One of these causes is caste, which is an important institution.

This community's socio-economic level is very low, and it is lower than the socio-economic level of other caste groups in the state. Hadis are not in a financial position to be able to afford the cost of private medical care. However, because public health care services are not readily available to them, they are coerced into gaining access to and making use of private health care services. A couple of the replies, on the other hand, demonstrate that there is also a level of ignorance among Hadis and that they do not inquire about the presence of or the availability of low-cost health care in the town.

According to a local RMP who has been working in the neighbourhood for a number of years now, both in the Muslim Mohalla and the Bauri Cooli, the government offers a number of perks, each of which takes a somewhat different shape, to those who choose to undergo permanent contraceptive techniques such as a vasectomy or tubectomy. However, the provision of monetary advantages does not currently entice a greater number of individuals than it formerly did some years ago. Even the monetary rewards that are gained are distributed among those who bring the patient to the hospital as well as those who are already there. A sub divisional hospital may be found in the Bokaro district. not a hospital serving a district (Zila). Patients who are going to have permanent contraceptive treatments done on them are transported to Bokaro General Hospital (BGH), which is a well-equipped facility that is supported by Bokaro Steel Plant. The phrase "health for all" is not the most important consideration; rather, it is important to determine who is eligible for benefits and what segments of the population have access to and can make use of this programme.

Vasectomy is not a widely practised form of birth control in Hadi communities. If questions concerning family planning services were posed to anyone from this group, it is safe to assume that they would give the impression of being terrified and more frightened.

In order to get to the bottom of things, one needs to look at the data that was provided by the respondents in addition to the secondary sources.

The main healthcare facility (PHC) in Chas town is responsible for the care of the Hadi Cooli. There is one Auxiliary Nurse Midwife (A NM) appointed to visit the location where the field work is being done, which is about three kilometres away. This area is about in the middle of the study. Another primary health care facility, known as Cheera Chas, can be found at the opposite end of the town and is about the same distance away. However, Cheera Chas was founded in order to serve the vast majority of the rural population as well as the villages that are next to it and are located in the immediate proximity of the market and the town area. This primary health care provider prepares the medical records for the family planning services, which are then forwarded to the Chas primary health care provider for final documentation. The target method is still used, which is accepted by the ANMs, despite the fact that they do not have any papers of this kind.

There are provisions that ANM/BHW will visit the residences in order to make the services more accessible to the general public. Within this neighbourhood, ANM/BHW personnel have gone to the homes of 18 responders, but the other homes have not been checked out.

Table 5.5 Visit of ANMs/BHWs

Serial No	Respondents' Response	Male	Female	Total
1	Yes	13	5	**18**
2	No	12	8	**20**
	Total	**25**	**13**	**38**

First, one of the reasons mentioned by health staff for the low number of house visits is that the PHC is situated in a remote area compared to Hadi Cooli. Second, the families do not go to the health centre in order to acquire treatments for free or at a reduced cost because of the distance, as well as for an excessive number of other reasons, which are covered in the various chapters. In this setting, the requirement of ANM/BHW visiting the residences of the Hadi community becomes increasingly vital; yet, the visits alone are not sufficient to meet what is eventually required by this group and are less than required. Access to the Hadi Cooli was made difficult for those from outside the community as a result of the clogged, dirty, and open drains and discharge of water. Thirty-eight people filled out the survey, and thirteen men and five women stated that an ANM or BHW had visited them at some point. In a typical month, members of the medical staff were observed visiting patients and engaging with them. Twenty of those who replied did not agree, and some even gave a negative response. There were a total of twelve male respondents who indicated that no health workers or staff like to visit their house, and eight female respondents who displayed similar reactions. Of these twenty, the responses of the male and female respondents were almost the same.

In the community, the aforementioned replies were taken into consideration during the debate with members of various castes. Even during the discussion that took place among the members of the caste, people's sentiments remained consistent. Elders were of the idea that the bulk of the physicians and health officers belong to upper castes and, as a result, they wouldn't bother spending time in the untouchables' neighbourhood. This was due to the fact that the elders believed the upper castes were more prestigious. They appeared to have the mindset that upper castes would not feel sufficient sympathy even to send other health practitioners to the portions of society that were the poorest and weakest. In addition, the non-availability of medications has decreased the willingness of even the neediest and most impoverished families to attend health centres, as well as the mood of the poorest and most needy families. Simply going to the doctor to get their picture taken will not help them get well from their ailment.

Table 5.6 Child Immunised (Last birth)

Serial No	Immunisation	Number of children
1	DPT	18
2	Polio	14
3	Not immunised	6
	Total	**38**

Note: Table 5.6 shows immunisation of respondents' children at the last birth

In reference to the vaccination of children, the table (5.6) that can be found above displays the vaccines that were given to the respondents' most recently born kids. The respondents' most recent five births are all that will be used in the research.

The very concept of immunisation is something that Hadis have never encountered before in their existence. Getting immunised is critical for establishing resistance and fighting off future infections in the human body as well as in the bodies of animals and plants; however, the topic of discussion for immunity at this point will be limited to humans.

Therefore, it is highly vital and absolutely necessary to offer vaccination services to all children in order to protect subsequent generations. It is possible that there are some causal correlations between the health of a person in the Hadi group and the health of the general population of the town, and that these ties may represent the economic prosperity of the state. Examining a person's susceptibility to illness as well as their level of exposure to infectious and communicable illnesses is one of the best ways to get a better grasp on the intricate relationship between caste and health care in India.

If an individual is not immunised against any of the communicable illnesses, they are at risk of contracting at least one of the diseases that may be passed on to others. But those who are marginalised, those who are oppressed, and those who live in socioeconomic situations that are less favourable are the most susceptible to harm. These people are mostly Dalits, women, and children. The youngsters living in the Hadi colony are particularly vulnerable, as the table to your right demonstrates.

Eighteen of the most recent births (out of a total of 38 children) received a dosage of DPT, and 14 of the youngsters were immunised against polio and other diseases. As can be seen in the chart, the other six youngsters did not receive their vaccinations. The proliferation of smaller hospitals and clinics that are administered by private businesses is one factor that is causing the current scenario to evolve. Patients from every caste and group, irrespective of discrimination and socioeconomic distance, are drawn to private hospitals as a result of the intensive marketing that is conducted by these facilities. It was generally accepted by Hadi scholars that vaccination was the primary means by which polio might be prevented. This demonstrates how intense the project was, yet nothing other than polio has such a significant existence in the memories of Hadis' lives or such an important role in their meaning. The "Tika," as it is known in the area (the word "Tika" is used for vaccination in Hindi), has gained popularity within the community; yet, why have the other vaccine campaigns failed or are nearly never utilised?

There was not a single responder who was aware of the programmes; instead, a dose of DPT or another immunisation is only administered to youngsters at the time of their regular medical visits. Through the time of the fieldwork, the number of polio cases was higher in certain areas of the Bokaro district; nevertheless, it was determined through a group discussion with the personnel at the health institution that these cases were not abruptly being reported among Hadis. There are fewer health care facilities available to the urban population in the more remote portions of the city or on the outside of the city. In some of the most distant and inner regions of the district, a small number of missionaries have set up health care facilities that are superior to those managed by the state. One of these organisations is called Asha Vihar, and it is located in the northwest corner of the district. It has a solid foundation and a well-developed infrastructure. They do not charge the families that have the lowest income, and even if they do, they only collect a small sum. This facility is mostly run by a German organisation (an NGO operating in the region to provide healthcare at very little cost), and a team of specialists from Germany travels here to treat children who have been affected by polio. However, those living in the surrounding rural regions are the only ones who can visit this centre; those living in the city are excluded. When we compare the relationships between the medical personnel working in public health care centres and other private hospitals, we find that their attitudes and behaviours towards patients are vastly different from one another. Patients have observed that private health care displays a positive attitude and has empathy for the conditions they are suffering from.

The majority of respondents gave unfavourable responses when asked about Hadis' relations with health care providers who visit their settlement. These responses were in response to a question about the ties of Hadis with health care providers. There are virtually no households that can point to positive interactions with, positive recollections of, or positive relations with members of the healthcare workforce. Due to the fact that most births take place in the comfort of the mother's own home, hospitals and other medical facilities do not receive every newborn baby. PHCs point to their limited resources as the reason they are unable to offer medical care to all of the underserved populations. Caste is the single most significant barrier that stands in the way of Dalit people having access to health care services, notwithstanding all of the other reasons that exist.

Table 5.7 Family Planning Services availed

Serial No	Respondent	Antenatal / Postnatal care availed				Total
		Iron folic	Anti tetanus	Post natal	None	
1	Male	1	11	1	12	25
2	Female	1	4	0	8	13
	Total	2	15	1	20	38

Note: "Male" respondents who spoke about female family members

The prenatal care that was received by female respondents as well as by the wives of male respondents is detailed in Table 5.7. Only one of the total of thirty-eight individuals received postnatal care, while two received iron folic, fifteen had tetanus vaccinations, and the total number was thirty-eight. It was clear that not a single woman in Chas had visited the public health clinic because not a single one of the female respondents who had spoken at the time of the interview had asked about the specifics of this service. Since Chas PHC does not have the infrastructure necessary to provide these treatments in an appropriate manner, your only other choice is to go to Bokaro General Hospital of the BSL. Because the prices that are paid to non-workers at the Bokaro Steel Plant are far greater than the rates that are charged to employees, it might be difficult to afford treatment. One of the female respondents had gotten iron folic acid, and four of the female respondents had received the anti-tetanus vaccination. Postnatal care was not provided to any of them. This means that the RMPs have the potential to earn more money. In circumstances like these, the financial value of the spiritual support and medical counselling that are made accessible to the families is difficult to ascertain because very few costs are incurred. All of the RMPs reside in the surrounding communities, so they are never reluctant to respond to emergencies, even at ungodly hours. When they treat patients at a lower cost and attend to them during inconvenient hours, this helps their clinics become more established and bring in more people. According to one of the RMPs, "we try to do anything for the delivery cases at home, even if it means conducting occasional small experiments." If these life-threatening instances can be treated, the faith of the patient's family and neighbours will grow, in addition to the larger and more lucrative amounts that will be given to us.

During the course of the inquiry that took place at the Hadi Cooli, one member of the Bauri caste stood out and deserves to be mentioned in this paragraph. This information was provided by the RMP, which eventually prevailed in their efforts to oversee the delivery of a challenging case. He arrived at the scene (one patient in a family in his area) at midnight when the family called on him amid intense delivery pains since it was not feasible to send the mother to a nursing home. The case included one patient in the family. The members of the family pleaded with him to assist and treat the pregnant woman in order to facilitate a risk-free birth to the very best of his abilities. If he hadn't taken the chance, the RMP would have lost the trust of that family and the other people in the neighbourhood. He administered three vials of glucose to the labouring mother, as well as any other necessary medications, by injection.

Home settings accounted for the vast majority of births. Within the Dalit community, traditional Dais were accorded greater rank and more respect as a result of the important role they played in childbirth. In the event of an emergency, however, the local RMPs are quickly contacted in order to provide additional medical care. RMPs have the possibility of making more money given the dangers of treating women in severe delivery situations. The newborns and the reliance of the families are also greater, owing to the availability of the RMPs whenever needed. Finally, after many long hours of waiting and struggling for the pregnant woman, she gave birth to a healthy baby who survived and was in good health the next morning. This was the first morning after the mother had given birth. This took all of his expertise and cost him the faith of the entire caste group, but the successful delivery gave him a handsome amount and increased both faith and rapport on his shoulders. However, his failure to deliver caused him to lose the faith of the entire caste group.

In a word, the purpose of this chapter is to assess the level of wellbeing among the Hadi community. It investigates the various problems and features of Dalit health, focusing mostly on the populations that work in dirty and "polluted" jobs.

The special situation of Hadis, in terms of their health problems and the usage of health care facilities, would inevitably be distinct from that of other caste groups located inside the state. This socioeconomic group's urban upbringing does not contribute to an improvement in the accessibility or utilisation of health care services because of the nature of the urban environment in which they live.

CHAPTER FIVE

BEST PRACTICES – FINDINGS AND CONCLUSION

In this study, "Dalit" alludes to those deprived, segregated, marginalised, and considered primitive and untouchable across religious and regional lines. The urban Dalit population relies on dirty and menial traditional occupations as their primary source of income and family support. In contrast, the rural population in the state of Jharkhand does feel the existence of vast mineral and natural resources; however, a large number of the rural family population is forced to depend on the small land that does not produce enough crop to feed the families when they could have been given the chance to work in factories, industrial units, and the mineral sector to earn a living wage. Numerous families are compelled to abandon rural areas because natural mineral resources have become the focus of development for the wealthy and state-owned production facilities. This is a unique aspect of the disparity between the benefits available to Dalits in the state and how severely they are impacted by restricted access to immense resources. Dalits are excluded from the larger social structure due to their inability to access minerals and agricultural land and their near-total lack of government employment. The Dalits in the state of Jharkhand are distinct from those in the neighbouring state of Bihar because of their traditional exclusionary axis. Most of the Dalit population comprises Jharkhand residents who do not own property or state resources.

Health care services are nothing more than a distant notion in their wretched existence. The socioeconomic situation has prevented Dalits from focusing on their right to fundamental health and educational facilities for all impoverished Hadi caste children. The decline in public health care services is not due to caste, socioeconomic status, etc. However, the decline in the structural level of health centres and the quality of health care delivery has significantly impacted and contributed to the state's declining service utilisation.

Through social mobilisation, it must be ensured that Dalits are aware of the unjust nature of the sociopolitical inequalities in which they find themselves in order to prepare them to fight for the implementation of their rights in all spheres, including the availability of high-quality health services. Manual scavenging has been practised, but providing aid to the community is not society's or the government's top priority. During the research period, the direct management of night soils and carcases is replaced by using a few instruments. Few residential communities have drainage systems, while the overwhelming majority of homes have septic containers for sewage disposal.

In the preceding segments of the dissertation, issues pertinent to Dalit health have been extensively and empirically highlighted to provide context for the analysis. This is one of the first studies on the Hadi caste, who reside primarily in Jharkhand, West Bengal, and Odisha.

In the study area, there are 690 females per 1000 males among the Hadis (a Dalit community), whereas the Bokaro district has 895 females per 1000 males (Census of India, 2001). This reflects the low sex ratio of women and their declining socioeconomic and social status in the city. There are a variety of causes for this, but poverty, illiteracy, and cultural factors will be examined more closely in future research.

Also, the literacy rate among Hadis is extremely low, particularly among women. Extreme poverty among Hadi caste families directly impacts women's health, according to the study. In comparison to other categories, the low sex ratio among females demonstrates illiteracy and a lack of social awareness. This causes and contributes to higher rates of mortality and morbidity. The respondents' rates of literacy are very low. Table 4.5 reveals that out of 198 respondents, the largest group is illiterate (87). In contrast, the second-largest group (72) did not attain the primary level of schooling available to other castes in the Hadi Cooli settlement neighbourhood. 1 instruction.

It is possible to determine the intriguing relationship between women's education and maternal mortality. Women constituted only 13 of the total 38 respondents. No female respondent attained a primary education or had the opportunity to pursue higher levels of education. In general, minimal levels of educational attainment are highly prevalent. Women and men require comparable healthcare services, but reproductive healthcare requires special attention for women. Women are more likely to be archaic, impoverished, and have a lower educational and health status. Table 4.5 demonstrates that illiteracy characterises the largest group of women who never attended school or received any education. Remarkably, none of the thirteen women selected for the study had any level of education.

Hadis are categorised into four income categories using the same method for locating respondents' annual income groups. The majority of the population has an annual income of less than ten thousand rupees. Approximately fifty per cent of respondents earn less than ten thousand dollars, followed by thirty-six per cent who earn between ten and twenty thousand. According to the available evidence, most of the Hadi population belongs to inferior socioeconomic classes. This is reflected in the form of the dwelling Hadis owns. The majority of the population has its own home because they have lived in the area for generations, but kutcha and semi-pucca dwellings are also prevalent. Bauri and Hadi Cooli, two Dalit settlements in Chas, primarily comprise earthen huts (Kutcha), demonstrating the destitution of Dalit households.

Considering the number of accommodations available per individual, the socioeconomic reflection demonstrates the disadvantageous conditions of Dalits. Overcrowding and congestion have undeniable effects on the health of individuals. The average number of guests per room is 5.21 per cent, which is extremely difficult to comprehend. The lack of culinary space within a home heightens its inhabitants' susceptibility. Generally, the majority of families cook food outside their front entrance.

Because there is no effective drainage system, the environment encircling the settlement (Cooli and Mohalla) is unclean. Nearly fifty per cent of respondents lacked any drain, while the remainder had open spaces or drainage. The area needs more infrastructure. Even in the not-too-distant future, their capacity to provide each residence with its source of potable water needs to be increased. In contrast to many other communities that have installed their water sources at astronomical costs, hand pumps and bore water are unattainable for them. Therefore, they obtain water from a public faucet in the market area, approximately one kilometre away. Only two households have alternative water sources; the remainder relies on public faucets. Comprehending the Hadi community's context will be simpler if we relate the housing condition to the source of potable water and household income.

Morbidity is a crucial indicator for determining any individual's or community's health, but it isn't easy to measure. The relationship between household socioeconomic characteristics and morbidity is reflected in the study population. This contributes to the study of the morbidity, or illness, of the larger community. Nevertheless, the morbidity pattern is restricted to the respondents.

In terms of the total number of cases, tuberculosis has a high prevalence. Twelve instances of skin disease were discovered, whereas only ten cases of tuberculosis were discovered. This pertains to occupations requiring unclean work, such as accessing manholes, which carry a high risk of infections such as tuberculosis, skin diseases, etc. Six males had tuberculosis, which is extremely prevalent among those who scour and scavenged. This association is strengthened when associated with cold and respiratory symptoms. There may be cough sufferers who have not undergone a sputum test or other examination. Asthma is more prevalent among individuals engaged in scouring and scavenging.

I want to add one more point: why are fever cases even higher among male respondents engaged in scouring and scavenging than among manual labourers, rickshaw pullers, and other occupations?

Female respondents reported similar circumstances. 75% of instances are identified among female respondents who are engaged in sweeping and scavenging. There appears to be a correlation between asthma, the common cold, congestion, and skin diseases.

Morbidity, with a focus on reproductive and infant health care utilisation, is primarily viewed in terms of health care utilisation. Family planning services are utilised by only approximately 34% of the study population. In this number, women are underrepresented. Two out of thirteen women were able to access family planning services, or approximately 15 per cent.

The utilisation of health care services is influenced by a variety of factors, including community literacy, political participation, and economic prosperity, among others. However, cultural factors also play a significant role in determining health status and health service utilisation.

The lack of interaction with health personnel or Auxiliary Nurse Midwives contributes to the decline in the utilisation of health services and the low quality of health services. As shown in Table 5.6, only 47 per cent of respondents report visits from an ANM or BHW. ANM must take pregnant women in the population into account. Most births are attended by traditional birth attendants called Dais, who are assisted by local RMPs. After an intensive campaign for polio eradication, immunisation grew in popularity. Still, caste-based social distance and occupational impropriety in the eyes of upper castes have hindered Dalit immunisation and contributed to a decline in access to healthcare. The burden of Dalit identity as one of the lowest-ranking castes in the Indian caste structure has increased the severity of exclusion and discrimination. This is because being lower on the caste hierarchy and being associated with menial occupations demonstrates their position in the caste hierarchy and occupation. In addition, high-caste healthcare personnel do not like handling the bodies of patients from low-caste families, thereby contributing to further deprivation in terms of healthcare accessibility. Touching lower caste members will increase the empathy of upper caste health personnel and increase the likelihood of interaction, but it does not guarantee enhanced access to health care. There is no prospect for a democratic society to have a respectful doctor-patient relationship or an empathic relationship between medical staff and Hadi caste patients.

As shown in Table 5.8 on antenatal and postnatal care, the situation is very poor: only two respondents had access to Reproductive and Child Health (RCH) services at the primary health care (PHC) facility in Chas, while five cases of anti-tetanus and postnatal infections were reported. The field data also suggests that cultural beliefs, taboos, social norms, practises, and social values all play significant roles in shaping the trend of healthcare service utilisation and accessibility.

The health infrastructure includes four criteria: accessibility, availability, cultural and social acceptability, and affordability for the majority of people, particularly those of lower socioeconomic classes and strata. Caste is a significant barrier to the accessibility and availability of healthcare services.

Caste plays an essential role in shaping an individual's conduct, particularly in regard to service utilisation. The utilisation of health care services is determined by a person's social standing in society. Accessibility is determined by the decision and propensity of the individual seeking care and the care providers' willingness to reach out to those in need.

The derogatory and inhumane conduct of the staff undermines the confidence and self-esteem of the individuals and places them in a state of existential crisis. The state of Jharkhand has failed to provide benefits to impoverished families native to the state, and it appears that the sociopolitical conditions that have governed the state for over two decades are no longer relevant. They have reached a point where it is necessary to depart from their constitutional obligation to provide equal access and fundamental amenities. Decades have passed since the concept of a right to life and dignity was reinstated. The only political proposal to be presented was the 1993 passage of the law prohibiting manual scavenging by the Indian parliament. In numerous regions of the nation's territory, scavenging is unparalleled. The current discussion on the health of Dalits is not limited to the marginalised Hadi caste that practises manual scavenging in slightly modified forms and methods. The problem of Dalits, particularly communities living with caste-based traditional occupations, has received scant attention in the sociological literature of India before the early 1990s, except for a few studies. There is a need to contextualise sociological understandings of health and illness in the context of a Dalit community and link them to sociological perspectives on health and illness.

Additionally, it is necessary to pose questions that can enhance the learning and employment of the impoverished. Are the health care service provider's actions solely following exclusionary practices and a hindrance to a community seeking better and more affordable public health care? The Indian constitution requires the state to provide a bare minimum of essential educational and health services, not as a luxury but as a fundamental privilege for all citizens. In Jharkhand, Dalits are second only to Adivasis in demand for manual labour and menial employment. Caste-based prohibitions and sanctions prohibiting the choice of occupations other than those ascribed by birth to a caste This has resulted in segregation, and caste is the primary reason for less use of health care services among the studied population.

Best practices are not limited to the birth status of Dalit communities in India and their sociocultural positioning within the existing social structure. It is also essential to comprehend the relationship between social status and occupation, exclusion from health care and education, and lack of access to public spaces. Regardless of the caste and religious heritage of the families and patients, the constitution of India mandates that certain elements be present and facilitate equal access to and use of health care services for all citizens. In this context, caste is one of the most significant barriers to healthcare services in a small municipality and could effectively resolve issues of exclusion and discrimination. The sociological significance of health within a community facilitates understanding the social relationship and dynamics between Dalits and upper castes in health institutions.

Modern society and nation must query the framework of citizenship, founded solely on an individual's birth and not on affiliation with any caste or creed. How India portrays herself as a modern nation and society, based on the historical foundations upon which it is founded and an investigation into the practices of equity in health care availability, is never possible. It requires significant consideration in the policy-making process of the state. As a new state, Jharkhand must ensure that impoverished communities, such as the Hadi caste, have access to quality healthcare and the right to health. The study does not represent the state as a whole; rather, it focuses on a specific town and is based on an empirical study of traditional low-caste settlements performing menial and manual scavenging for over two centuries, as evidenced by field data. The present description in the entire text relates only to one social group engaged in menial and lowly-ranked occupations, and the author has been unable to convert or transfer the analysis to other occupations. The entire field data and narrative investigation relied on sociological methodologies from the sociology of health, which examined the social interaction between societies in and of themselves and health. The interactions between patients and physicians or practitioners do not occur in isolation but within a tightly-knit social structure. In light of this, the book poses the question of how morbidity and mortality affect social life and vice versa. The dominant social practices of a given society similarly determine the social structure of public and private healthcare systems. For the state to enhance public health centres, a significant portion of the health budget must be allocated (Akram, 2014). The chapters on these pages have examined the social interactions between professionals and patients at various levels of treatment, as well as the reality of caste discrimination in accessing health care services in India. Despite the state's enormous economic prosperity and development, the promises made to every citizen regarding health and education still need to be fulfilled. Each successive government has destroyed the families' hope, and none of the families in this community has found a new lease on life through alternative occupations. A profession that provides families prosperity and respect is still a dream to the Hadi caste and similar other castes suffering discrimination and exclusion.

BIBLIOGRAPHY

Akram, Mohammad. (2014). Maternal *Health in India: Contemporary Issues and Challenges*. Jaipur: Rawat Publications.

Anand, Dinesh. S. (2000). *Who is a Sudra.* New Delhi: Blue Moon Books.

Bader, M.D.M., Warkentien, S. (2016). 'The Fragmented Evolution of Racial Integration since the Civil Rights Movement. *Sociological Science*, March 2, 2016.

Bandyapadhyay, Mridula and MacPherson, S. (1998). "*Women and Health: Tradition and Culture in Rural India.*" Aldershot: Ashgate Publishing.

Bendix, R., and Lipset, S.M. (1996). "*Class, Status and Power.*" New York: Free Press.

Beteille, A. (1997). *"Inequality among Men."* New Delhi: Oxford University Press, P.3-25.

George, M. (2014). Voice of Illness and Voice of Medicine in Doctor-Patient Interaction. In Madhu Nagla (Ed.), *Sociology of Health*, Vol. 4. New Delhi: Sage Publications India Pvt Ltd.

Hutton, J.H. (1963). *Caste in India: Its Nature, Function and Origin." Oxford*: Oxford University Press.

Ilaiah, K. (1996). *Why I Am Not Hindu.* Calcutta: SAMYA Publications.

Jan C.M. (1999). *Women Helping Themselves to Health: the Experience of Jan Chetna Manch."* Chandankiyari, Bokaro.

Jones, L.J. (1998). "*The Social Context of Health and Health Work.*" London: Macmillan Publishers Limited.

Kalelkar, K. (1955). "*First Backward Classes Commission.*" New Delhi: Government of India.

Kamble, M.D. (1982). *"The Scheduled Castes."* New Delhi: Ashish Publishing House.

Karkal, M. (2000). "Poverty, Health and Nutrition." Paper Prepared for NGO Academic Paper for WDR. New Delhi.

Lal, S. (1999). "*The Changing Bhangis of India: A Study of Castse Association.*" Jaipur: Sublime Publications.

Luders, J.E. (2010). *The Civil Rights Movement and the Logic of Change.* New York: Cambridge University Press.

Marriott, M. (1973). "Caste Systems." In Chicago: *Encyclopedia of Britannica*. Vol. 3; Pp 982-91. Chicago: Encyclopedia Britannica.

Marx, K., and Davis, R. (1994). "*A Contribution to the Critique of Hegel's Philosophy of Right: Introduction.*" In J. O'Malley (Ed.), *Marx: Early*

Political Writings (Cambridge Texts in the History of Political Thought, pp. 57-70). Cambridge: Cambridge University Press. doi:10.1017/CBO9781139168007.007

Massey, J. (1997). "*Downtrodden: The Struggle of India's Dalits for Identity, Solidarity and Liberation.*" Geneva: World Council of Churches.

Moon, V. (1989). "*Writing and Speeches of Bhim Rao Ambedkar (WSBRA).*" Vol. 5, Education Department, Government of Maharashtra.

Nagla, M (Ed.). (2014). *Sociology of Health*, Vol. 4. New Delhi: Sage Publications India Pvt Ltd.

Nandkarni, M.V. (1997). "Broadcasting Process in India and Dalits." *Economic and Political Weekly*, Aug 16.

National Health Policy. (2001). "*Legitimising Privatisation*", New Delhi: Delhi Science Forum.

Park, J.E. and Park, K. (1991). "*Textbook of Preventive and Social Medicine.*" Jabalpur: Banarsidas Bhanot Publishers.

Parvathamma, C. (1989). "*Scheduled Castes at the Crossroads.*" New Delhi: Ashish Publishing House.

Pathak, B. (1991). "*Road to Freedom: A Sociological Study on the Abolition of Scavenging in India.*" New Delhi: Motilal Banarsidass Publications.

Prasad, J. (1996). "*Equality versus Justice: The Problem of Reservations for Backward Classes.*" New Delhi: Deep and Deep Publications.

Prasad, P. 2014. Narratives of Sickness and Suffering: A study of Malaria in South Gujarat. In Madhu Nagla (Ed.), *Sociology of Health*, Vol. 4. New Delhi: Sage Publications India Pvt Ltd.

Qadeer, I., Sen K., and Nayar, K.R. (2002) "*Public Health and the Poverty of Reforms: The South Asian Predicament.*" (Ed.) New Delhi: Sage Publications.

Rama, S. (1995). "*Scavengers in Indian Society.*" New Delhi: M D Publications.

Ravindran, T.K.S. (1996). "Social Inequality and Child Health Status: A Study of a Scheduled Caste Population." In "*Health, Poverty and Development in India,*" edited by Monica Das Gupta, Lincoln C. Chen and T.N. Krishnan. New Delhi: Oxford University Press.

Rawat, H. (1999). "*Encyclopaedia of Sociology.*" Jaipur: Rawat Publications.

Shah, G. (2002). "*Dalits and States: An overview.*" (Ed.). New Delhi: Concept Publishing Company.

Shah, G. (1990). "*Social Movement in India.*" New Delhi: Sage Publications. Pp. 17-20.

Shah, G. (1997). "*Caste: Its Twentieth Century Avatar.*" New Delhi:

Penguin Books India (p) Ltd.

Shah, G. (2001). "*Dalit: Identity and Politics*." New Delhi: Sage Publications.

Sharma, K.L. (1997). "Caste and Class in the Emergence of Dalit Identity and Movement." *The Administrator*, Vol. XLII, Jan-March 35-53.

Singh, S. (1980). "*Socio-economic Conditions of SC in India*." Allahabad: Progressive Book Depot.

Srinivas, M.N. (1952). "*Religion and Society among the Coorgs of South India*." Oxford: Clarendon Press.

Srinivasan, N.R. (1998). "*Socio-Economic Study of Bokaro*." Steel Authority of India Ltd., Bokaro Steel Plant, Bokaro Steel City, p.48.

Srivastava, B.N. (1997). "*Manual Scavenging in India: A Disgrace to the Country*." New Delhi: Concept Publishing Company.

Teltumde, A. (1998). "Impact of Economic Reforms on Dalits in India." A paper presented in the seminar on "Economic Reform and Dalits in India," organised by the University of Oxford, UK.

The New Encylclopaedia Britannica. (1997). "*Macropaedia*." William Benton Publisher, Chicago. USA, Vol. 3.

Thorat, S.K. and Deshpande R.S. (2001). "*Caste System and Economic Inequality: Economic Theory Evidence*." In Ghanshyam Shah (ed.) '*Dalit Identity and Politics*', edited by Ghanshyam Shah, 46-49. New Delhi: Sage Publication. Pp 46-49.

Webster, C.B. (1994). "*The Dalit Christians: A History*." Delhi: Indian Society for Promoting Christian Knowledge.

Ziyauddin, K. M. and Kasi, E. (2009). "Dimensions of Social Exclusion: Ethnographic Explorations." Newcastle-upon-Tyne: Cambridge Scholars Publishing.

Ziyauddin, K.M. (2012). "*Muslim Scavengers in India: Perception and Perspectives of Social Exclusion*." Germany: LAMBERT Academic Publishing.

Zurbrigg, S. (1984). "*Rakku's Story: Structure of Ill Health and the Source of Change*." Bangalore: Centre for Social Action.

Sulabh International Social Service Organisation. (2001). "Scavengers: No More Untouchables." New Delhi.